Life after Kids

Life after Kids

Rediscover Yourself and Thrive Beyond Motherhood

Brooke Stillwell and
Lynne Mouw

JB JOSSEY-BASS™

A Wiley Brand

Published by John Wiley & Sons, Inc., Hoboken, New Jersey.
Published simultaneously in Canada.

ISBNs: 9781394295340 (hardback), 9781394295364 (epdf), 9781394295357 (epub)

For general information on our other products and services or for technical support, please contact our Customer Care Department within the United States at (800) 762-2974, outside the United States at (317) 572-3993 or fax (317) 572-4002.

Wiley also publishes its books in a variety of electronic formats. Some content that appears in print may not be available in electronic formats. For more information about Wiley products, visit our web site at www.wiley.com.

Library of Congress Cataloging-in-Publication Data

Names: Stillwell, Brooke author | Mouw, Lynne author
Title: Life after kids : rediscover yourself and thrive beyond motherhood / Brooke Stillwell and Lynne Mouw.
Description: Hoboken, New Jersey : Jossey-Bass, [2025] | Includes bibliographical references.
Identifiers: LCCN 2025021750 (print) | LCCN 2025021751 (ebook) | ISBN 9781394295340 cloth | ISBN 9781394295364 adobe pdf | ISBN 9781394295357 epub
Subjects: LCSH: Motherhood | Parent and adult child | Self-actualization (Psychology) in women
Classification: LCC HQ759 .S6946 2025 (print) | LCC HQ759 (ebook) | DDC 306.874/3—dc23/eng/20250613
LC record available at https://lccn.loc.gov/2025021750
LC ebook record available at https://lccn.loc.gov/2025021751

Cover Design: Paul McCarthy
Cover Art: © Getty Images | Malerapaso
Printed and bound by CPI Group (UK) Ltd, Croydon, CR0 4YY

C9781394295340_080825

Contents

Acknowledgments

Dr. Brooke

Before I thank anyone else, I have to start by thanking the one person that has been with me from the very beginning of Life after Kids. From the time of its inception during that New Hampshire hike several years ago, Lynne and I have been walking alongside each other to build and support this fabulous community of midlife women. We've worked tirelessly. We've had fun, shed tears, and yes, even had some major fights. Lynne has been by my side every step of the way for over 20 years. Our friendship has stood the arduous test of time and has seen us through graduations, careers, marriage, childbirth, loss, raising kids, and some pretty fabulous travel. Life after Kids is a testament to what is possible when two very different women come together and share a common goal of making the world a teeny bit better than the way they found it even if they pull each other's hair out and cause just a few more gray hairs along the way. Lynne, none of this, including our book, would have been possible without your brilliant mind, and

I am so grateful to have had this roller coaster ride of a journey with you, my friend.

To Amy, Sophie, Christine, and the rest of the publishing team at Jossey Bass and Wiley, thank you for seeing something special in our work, for taking a chance on us, and for recognizing the many needs of a mom who's entering a new chapter of life. To Kim and the many peer editors that worked tirelessly on our book, thank you for making this book so much better than it originally was and for caring about it enough to cut through the pleasantries and tell it like it is. I appreciate you so very much. Without a doubt, you made my writing better.

To Candy, my friend and my sister, I don't even know where to begin. You have been instrumental in the launch of this book and getting it out into the world. Thank you for taking a seemingly overwhelming task and making it so much more manageable. I can't thank you enough for the difference you've made in my life both professionally and personally. Your ability to always show up with integrity and authenticity constantly astounds me. Without a doubt, my life is fuller because you are in it. Thank you for pushing me to be the best version of myself and challenging me in ways I didn't even know I needed.

To my three handsome, hilarious, and intelligent sons, Anthony, Andrew, and AJ, you are the reason for everything I do. My sun rises and sets on you and I cannot wait to see the wonderful ways in which you will make your way in this world. Thank you for making me a mom. Thank you for teaching me patience and what unconditional love really means. Thank you for making me a better person. Most importantly, thank you for giving me content for this book. *Life after Kids* would surely not have happened without you. I pray that the way I live my life daily is teaching you how to dream big for your own life and to know that anything is possible.

To my husband, Ken, I'm not sure if I should be writing you a thank you or an apology! When I'm in a zone, whether of writing or other work, I can be a bear, especially to you. Thank you for putting up with me. I am sorry for the things I said and did when

I was up at 12 am writing this book when I really needed to be sleeping! Through almost 25 years of marriage you have been my rock and my true north. You are my home. The things we've accomplished together this far in our life never cease to amaze me and I can't wait to see what the future holds for us. I would not be here without you loving me, challenging me, and yes, even calling me on my own BS. Thank you for keeping it real and for supporting me, encouraging me, and loving me through the writing of this book and the building of Life after Kids.

And finally and most importantly, I have to give all glory and praise to God. My fervent prayer over the last 20 years of my life has been that the Lord would open the right doors for my life, close the wrong doors, and give me the strength and discernment to walk through or away from each. I have been nothing less than blown away by the answers I've received from this prayer, the writing of this book included. Thank you, Jesus. Everything I am and all that I have done or ever will do is because of you.

Dr. Lynne

Of all of the writing I've done for this book, I've been the most excited to pen these acknowledgments. Yet, as I sit here to write it feels impossibly difficult to put into words my gratitude and love for each person who has contributed their time and talents to help us get to this point in our journey.

Most of all I want to thank my husband, Dr. Mark Mouw. Your unending love and acceptance leaves me humbled and feeling incredibly blessed every single day. There is no one more deserving of unconditional love than you because you so freely give it back to us. Thank you for being so patient and for always seeing something greater in me than I could see for myself. I'm easily the luckiest woman on earth because you are by my side and you still take my breath away all of these years later.

To Brooke, our friendship means the world to me. No matter the circumstances, I will always trust that we can find a path through the challenges together. Building this business with you has brought me more joy and healed my spirit in more ways than I could have ever imagined. None of it would have happened without you. You are the machine that drives Life after Kids. Thank you for making me laugh harder than anyone I know, thank you for taking the time to understand my strengths and thank you for just being you. I love you, friend.

To our editors and the publishing staff at Jossey Bass and Wiley, thank you for your guidance and your expertise in bringing this book to fruition. Without you all, we most certainly would not be here.

To my children, Lila and Dr. Jordan Mouw. Everything I am, I owe to the lessons you have both taught me. Jordan, I am eternally grateful for you coming into my life when you did. I'll always be in awe of how open and loving you were from the first moment we met. One of the greatest moments of my life was our mother-son dance at your wedding. I am endlessly proud of the man you are and the father you have become. To Jordan, Jamie, and the four little J's, I love you all to the moon and back.

Lila, thank you for the patience and grace you've extended to me in the past year while writing this book. I am continually amazed by your confidence and your positively contagious enthusiasm for life. I am so honored to be your Mom. I cannot wait for all of the exciting things you have coming your way in the years to come. A big piece of my heart will leave with you when you move to Texas this fall. I love you so much, Bumper. Go do big things with your life; your Mom and Dad will always be cheering you on.

I am and have been well loved by many people who encourage me to live my life well and give more to others than you take, not the least of which are my mother, Betty, and sister, Paula, brother-in-law, Cory, and my nephews—aka the Kings—Cole and Chase. I think Pop would be proud, would he not?

There are so many people who have handed out advice, impacted or inspired a teaching, or have mentored me along the way, too many to name but hopefully you know who you are.

A big thank you to my biweekly accountability girls: Wendy, Camilla, and Debbie. I am deeply appreciative of your friendship and counsel. It's amazing what's possible when a group of women commit to show up regularly for each other. To Tom, and Sue, thank you for loving me like a daughter and for giving me the greatest man to partner with. To Holly, thanks for keeping me sane in Iowa and always laughing. Your friendship has meant more to me than you know. Merily, thank you for regularly checking in and for helping me feel accepted just as I am. We are total opposites and a testament to how understanding your strengths just makes friendships better.

Finally, to all of the women in the Life after Kids community. Without you, none of this would be possible. Thank you for not accepting a life any less than the exciting and purpose-filled one you deserve. We thank you from the bottom of our hearts for supporting this book and for coming along with us on this journey.

About the Authors

Dr. Brooke Stillwell

Dr. Brooke Stillwell holds a doctorate degree in Chiropractic from Palmer College. She specializes in women's health and well-being and has been working with patients both chiropractically and nutritionally for over 20 years. She's extremely passionate about the health of moms and has founded and led wellness groups to help them flourish in their many roles.

She is also an author, speaker, co-host of the *Life after Kids* podcast, and co-founder of the Life after Kids community, where she reaches millions of moms globally who are seeking to live a meaningful life after their kids are grown. She and her husband, Ken, have raised three amazing young men and are currently living their best almost empty nest lives just outside of Boston with their doting fur babies, Bristol and London.

Dr. Lynne Mouw

In addition to her expertise as a Chiropractor and health and wellness expert for over 20 years, Dr. Lynne Mouw is a Certified Strengths and Enneagram coach. She is an author, key note speaker, co-host of the *Life after Kids* podcast and co-founder of the viral Life after Kids community. She is an aspiring DJ and dog lover. Mom to Lila and stepson Dr. Jordan Mouw, she is also a devoted "Gigi" to her four precious grandkids. She is committed to helping other women reach their potential by focusing them on what they do best. She and her husband, Dr. Mark Mouw, live just outside Omaha, Nebraska, but her happy place will always be overlooking the North Atlantic Ocean from a cliffside hiking trail in Newfoundland, Canada, where she was born and raised.

You can find the thriving Life after Kids Community on Instagram @life.afterkids. For more information, visit lifeafterkids.com.

Introduction

It was late summer 2021 and we were halfway down a mountain we'd just summited in Gilford, New Hampshire. We were moving at a pretty fast pace, and our conversation was keeping up with our feet. Maybe it was that we were at the end of the hike, we were at the end of the summer, or our kids were just about to head back to school, signaling we were one year closer to them leaving home, but whatever the case, our conversation turned to what we wanted our lives to look like in the next five to 10 years.

We were both chiropractors (we actually met almost 25 years ago in grad school), and we were ready to pivot away from working full time with patients in order to have more flexibility and time with our older kids. After all, the rate at which the days and years were flying by signaled we shouldn't take any time we have with our families for granted. Plus, we wanted to travel more, we wanted to do something together, and we wanted to use our experience with women—both in health and wellness and with the Gallup Strengths Finder tool as well as the Enneagram personality test—to make a difference in the world. But what could we do?

Over the course of our extensive friendship, we'd already experienced so many changes and life events. But one thing that never changed was our commitment to getting to know and understand ourselves better, to learn, to grow, to stay emotionally balanced, and to be as physically healthy as possible so that we could show up daily as our best selves. Now that our kids were growing up and we were staring down at empty nests, those things seemed even more important than ever because we knew we didn't just want to survive this phase of life; we wanted to thrive.

As we headed down the mountain, we came to a realization: If we were feeling this way about the thought of life beyond motherhood, surely other moms are, too. What if we started an online brand and community to connect moms in the same phase of life and to help them live a more fulfilling and meaningful life by finding new purpose, getting emotionally balanced and physically healthier, while also building friendships and connections?

And just like that, the Life after Kids community was born. Little did we know that as we took our last steps down the mountain on that hot August day having found new purpose and fulfillment for our life beyond motherhood, we were also taking our first steps toward helping thousands of other moms do the same. This book is the culmination of all the work, learning, and researching we've done, and the experiences we've had throughout our almost 25 years as friends and as well as health and wellness practitioners, and it includes every strategy, tip, and advice we've used with our patients, our coaching clients, and our online membership community.

Welcome to *Life after Kids*! We're so glad you're here.

Part I

PURPOSE

Chapter 1

It's Not About the Kids

By Dr. Brooke

In the Beginning: The Early Days of Motherhood

Twenty-one years seems like it should be a long time, yet I feel it blew right by me as if I was spinning around and around in circles outside on a bright sunny day as I used to do for fun as a little girl until I got so dizzy I couldn't walk straight, swiftly tumbling into the soft grass. That's exactly how I feel about motherhood—like I was spinning for fun at a dizzying speed, and when I stopped, I stumbled right into 2025.

How did I get here? I'd like to tell you I remember each day of motherhood clearly with the unparalleled ability to recall every sight, sound, scent, and feel of my children's younger years. But let me be perfectly honest: Most days, I was just trying to survive. In reality, a large portion of that time seems like a blur. Yet I can recall some moments as clearly as if I'm watching them take place on a 65-inch high-definition flat-screen TV, subtitles and all. Will you partake for a moment in one of the episodes with me?

It was a hot and sticky Monday in 2003, July 14 to be exact. Almost 10 days past due with my first pregnancy, I looked as if I'd swallowed a watermelon in one gulp; I was bursting at the seams, and I was exhausted not only from growing and carrying a human being around in my body for nine months but also from my dad asking me every 10 minutes how I felt and did I think labor would start soon. He also felt the need to shove a camera in my face for a picture directly after his repetitive interrogation.

Earlier that day, I had begun to feel tumultuous waves throughout my belly preparing my body for labor. As contractions began and then ramped up, I busied myself with what any other normal woman in labor with her first child would do. I watched a marathon of *Austin Powers* movies, while cooling and calming myself with Fudgsicles. When it was finally time to leave the house for hardcore labor to begin, I was disheveled and in moderate pain, face sticky and spackled with remnants of my chocolate dessert pacifier, wondering if I'd ever find my mojo again.

Let's be real for a moment, shall we? Nobody can prepare any of our hearts for what it feels like when our baby is placed in our arms for the first time. Regardless of how many books you read and classes you take, the reality is even better than the dream (until of course you bring said baby home and realize your life is never ever going to be the same and not always in a good way).

My first son finally came into the world during the wee hours of the morning of July 15. And once we got settled into our home, I quickly realized that life would never be the same. I distinctly remember my new parenting skills being put to the test one afternoon shortly after bringing Anthony home from the hospital. He was in a newborn rage, red-faced from his high-pitched screaming, and literally nothing I did could calm or quiet him. I sang, I swayed, I rocked, I swaddled, but nothing did the trick. Feeling helpless and way out of my league, I wondered why this little being didn't come with an owner's manual. In those moments, I recall thinking "life as I know it is over." I will never again be able to choose to cuddle up on the couch by myself in the quiet of my home on a lazy afternoon to watch a romantic comedy or a ridiculous reality show. My life was no longer my own.

Soon my new life, which really didn't belong to me anymore anyway, began to fly by. There were first birthdays, mommy and me classes, endless trips to the playground, play dates, two more births, preschool, sporting events, elementary school, nonstop carpooling, homework help, family vacations, middle school angst, and finally high school, first dates, and driver's ed. It was a whirlwind.

My life was a revolving door that just kept spinning. For more than 21 years, my life has been completely consumed with my children. They've grown my heart in ways I never guessed possible. They pushed me to be the best version of myself. They taught me patience and selflessness. Because of them I learned better time management and communication skills. They even just about single handedly built my social network as most of my friends were parents of their friends.

My kids are my greatest joy, sometimes my greatest heartache, and without a doubt my greatest teachers. And now as the revolving door begins to slow down for my exit into the next chapter of my life, I find that my kids are teaching me yet again, and this may be the biggest lesson yet: the art of letting go.

The Transition, the Lessons, and the Heartache of Motherhood

For most of us moms, from the time our first child comes into the world, there is a shift in our universe. Suddenly, our sun is rising and setting on them. The things that used to occupy our head space and require our time take a back seat to the needs of our children. Our needs become secondary to theirs. For example, you may get through a long and arduous week, wanting nothing more than to spend your Friday night soaking in a long hot bath with a good book or ordering a pizza and watching your favorite movie; instead, you spend your night at a youth basketball game. Maybe you planned a girls night out but had to cancel because there's no one to stay with the kids or your children need you to drive them somewhere. And, of course, there's nothing better than canceling that much needed appointment because as luck would have it, your child happens to get sick at the same time. Then one day, the youth sporting events are over, your children no longer need your supervision at home, and they start driving themselves everywhere they need to go.

The days of our children depending on us are indeed waxing and waning, and we're transitioning into life after kids. For much of our adult life, we put our own needs, hopes, and dreams on hold for our children to realize theirs, but now the door to our own life is opening again.

Perhaps we should feel excited about this. I mean for me, there was a time (as you'll recall from the previous section) that I grieved the loss of the ability to lay down on the couch and watch a movie by myself if so inclined. But ironically, now that life is granting me more freedom and I have the ability to watch said movie, I can't say that I'm over the moon excited about it. Can you relate?

If you're reading this book, I'm guessing you probably can. Ironically, we've hit midlife, our kids are grown or growing up, suddenly we have more freedom to do what we want and go where we want, but we feel lost and not sure what direction to even go. In a strange turn of events, the days of wishing we had just a few moments of peace and quiet to be by ourselves and collect our thoughts have led us to the peace and the quiet we craved, but now we're longing for the days of noise. To top it all off, we've traded the small worries we had for our kids like "Why won't they eat their vegetables" and "Will they ever learn to pee-pee on the potty" to "Will they choose the right life partner" and "Will they find a career that fulfills them." And don't get me started on the nights we lay in bed wondering if we did enough and whether or not we've prepared them well for life. Naturally, these circumstances can leave us feeling disconnected from life, a little lost, lonely, and even fearful.

If this sounds like you, take heart, because you are not alone. Our kids growing up and leaving home is a big deal and not something we need to "just get over." Dr. Lynne and I have been completely blown away by the response we've had to the Life after Kids community. So many women have shared with us the story of their older kids leaving home or preparing to leave, followed by the gaping hole left in their heart by the changes in their family dynamic. Others have thanked us for letting them know they're not alone in their feelings. Moms of college kids, military kids, traveling kids, trade school kids, and just older kids in general, all sharing one common denominator—their grief over saying goodbye to their kids' childhood knowing they won't get it back and the loneliness they feel since their kids left. Trust me when I say, I feel it, too.

When Your Child Leaves Home

My first son left for college in the fall of 2023, moving out of state to live on a campus that is a five-hour car ride away. Friends who had already been down this path tried to prepare me and related that the car ride home after dropping them off would be the worst. I was, however, completely blindsided by how gutted I felt when I walked in the door to my house without my son. Suddenly, my legs felt 10 times heavier than they actually were, and I struggled to put one foot in front of the other. I waded through my house as if I was walking in a swimming pool against the resistance of the water around me. My body and mind were utterly exhausted, much like I used to feel directly after taking an exam that I'd pulled an all-nighter for. I was at the end of my emotional rope. The waves of everything I'd been attempting to prepare my heart for all summer long suddenly came crashing down on me as the realization that my baby was no longer living in my home slapped me in the face with a splash so salty it made my eyes burn. I didn't try to ignore it. I didn't try to fight it. I didn't even cry, at least not at that moment. Instead, I did the only thing my body would allow me to do. I curled up on the couch with my bestie Bristol (she's a dog) and fell into a very sudden, deep, restful, and much needed nap.

The rest of the night proceeded without much drama. I had a nice dinner with my husband and my other two boys, relaxed for a bit, and then headed to bed. That's when the emotions rushed over me all over again. I was going to bed in my home, Anthony was no longer in his room, and he wouldn't be for quite some time. Here we go again with the drama. It's amazing the torture moms are capable of putting themselves through, especially when they lay down to go to bed at night. Eventually, the night led to morning, which led to the start of a new day. I'd love to tell you it was a fresh start, but the next day was only slightly better than the first. I just couldn't get past the hollow feeling I felt in the pit of my stomach, no matter how hard I tried to stay busy or distract myself.

That's exactly what I did in the months to follow. I kept myself very busy and distracted, throwing myself into the lives of my other boys, household chores, and work. Oh how grateful I was for my work. Slowly, as warm summer days turned to crisp autumn nights, my heart began to feel a little more whole again as long as I didn't attempt to go into Anthony's room (I kept that door shut).

Nonetheless, life was moving forward, and my nervous system began to feel more regulated, my brain a little more quiet. Texts, phone calls, and FaceTimes with Anthony helped tremendously. Hearing about his fun, growth, excitement, and new friends eased my mind. Before I knew it, fall break was upon us and Anthony was coming home! My momma's heart was so full in the days leading up to his arrival and so were my days as I eagerly cleaned the house, freshened his sheets, decorated for fall, and shopped for his favorite snacks and foods. I'll never forget him walking in the door that first day of break, how my heart skipped a beat, how the dogs pummeled him with excitement in our entryway, and how all felt right with the world once again.

Do you know what else I'll never forget? The day he left to go back to college again. We took him and his brothers out for a family dinner just before he left. Hugging and saying goodbye to him in the restaurant parking lot on that gloomy overcast evening broke my heart all over again. As I got in my own car and watched him drive off in his, the tears began to fall like the rain drops hitting my windshield, blurring my vision twice over. I arrived back home feeling particularly downtrodden and texted a mom friend who'd already been down this road to ask if my emotional uproar was normal and if the goodbyes would ever get easier. She assured me that she had been through the same, and what I was feeling was normal.

I think one of our Life after Kids community members said it best: "Having a kid in college is like the never-ending goodbye." Well said, my friend, well said. That first year of Anthony's college career was just as she stated. Every time I started getting used to him being gone, getting accustomed to the house being just a little bit empty and a lot more quiet, he'd come home and my heart would soar in spite of the mess, mounds of laundry, and extra cooking! But then he'd leave again, and I would feel as if I was right back where I started from. The goodbyes are always tough, especially in that first year.

Right Back Where We Started

Would you agree that in some ways, life after our kids are grown is just like being right back where we started? Let me clarify. Before we had kids, we were living a life of less responsibility, beholden to no one but ourselves and maybe our spouse/partner. We could come and go when we wanted, eat and cook what we wanted when we wanted, sleep in on the weekends if we felt like it, we didn't have to worry about sports or extracurricular activities, and we had so much time for self-care.

Then our children came along and all of that changed as suddenly their needs and schedules became more important than ours. Now that they're older with many or all of them out of the house, in some sense, we're back to life as we knew it before kids. Except for one BIG thing: Now we know what we're missing. We know what it's like to love another person more than ourselves. We know how it feels to have them sleeping safely under our roof at night and to check in with them over breakfast. We know how happy we feel when they walk through the door. And we are well aware of the joy we get when we hug them and tell them to be safe before they go to school or out with friends.

And once you know all these joys, you can't un-know them. For most moms, this phase of life with grown kids is not as simple as sucking it up and moving on knowing this was coming and that it's a normal part of life because the biggest piece of our heart is no longer near us most of the time. This is precisely why so many of us lament our kids leaving home and why we struggle in an empty nest. It's why we look through old photos with nostalgia and tears in our eyes. It's why we have a sense of foreboding every time we walk past their empty room. It's why we lay in bed at night thinking about them and looking forward to their next call, text, or FaceTime. And it's why we feel so lost and disconnected as we stare down and then enter an empty nest. Or is it?

Don't get me wrong: There is grief and mourning that comes with saying goodbye to your kids' childhood. I've experienced it myself, and I would never minimize the feelings. Plus, there's nothing like our kids growing up to smack us in the face with the harsh reality of how fleeting time is (except for maybe our own reflection in the mirror). But let me suggest that missing our kids, mourning their childhood, and getting older is not the only or even primary cause of why moms struggle so much with this phase of life. The real reason we have such difficulty navigating our kids growing up and leaving actually comes from within. It has everything to do with us and who we are, not our kids.

See, for most of our adult lives, we've identified as moms, and what we did was completely wrapped up in what our kids did. We lived life alongside them. For the most part, our life was their life. Who we were was seen in them. Of course, we'll never stop being a mom, and our kids will always need us to some extent. But now that they're grown, are independent, and have left or are leaving home, we stop and look around wondering who we are if we aren't mothering 24/7. We have an identity crisis of sorts. Our fears, our loneliness, our trepidation, and our disconnect comes from being uncertain with who we are in the world, how we fit in, and what we have to offer now that the kids are grown.

The Antidote for Living a Fulfilling Life Beyond Motherhood

Ironically, we have less responsibility, more freedom, and more choices for our life than we've had since our kids were born, but instead of looking at this as a new and exciting opportunity as we did when we were younger, we look around feeling lost and perhaps even irrelevant. Oh, but my friends, take heart because Dr. Lynne and I know the antidote, and we've been studying it for years. We don't need our kids to move back home. We don't need time to reverse. We certainly don't need to accept how we feel and lead a mediocre, less-than-fulfilling life.

Instead, we should take our feelings of loss, disconnection, loneliness, and irrelevancy and let them fuel the fire of change and growth. The antidote for our heartache is getting to know ourselves all over again and finding passion and purpose for our life. Moms of older kids need a reason, we need to be needed, we need a "why," and I hate to break it to you, but that "why" needs to be bigger than our kids.

If we wander haphazardly through the rest of our time here on Earth, centering our whole lives and beings around our kids, expecting them and their new life to be our primary source of joy, then our lives will never be as fulfilling and meaningful as they could be. Here are a few reasons why:

- Your kids will not always be happy in their life. Unfortunately, it's a fact. You and I have lived long enough to know that life is a tumultuous roller coaster ride, full of ups and downs. At one point or another, everybody struggles, and our kids will, too. We can no longer protect them in the same way we once did. They have to live their own lives, and while they'll always be our greatest joy, we have to find happiness outside of them.
- The happiest people in life focus on what they can control and let go of the things they can't. We can no longer control all of the decisions our kids make. We can't control their career path, whom they choose to marry, whether or not they have kids, and we certainly can't control where they decide to live. So let's not put our focus there.

Instead, let's focus on what we can control, things like how much time we make for our physical and emotional health, whom we want to build relationships with, where we want to live, and what we want to do with our day-to-day life.

I know that you want to live a second phase of life that is much more than mediocre. You wouldn't be reading this book if you didn't. And if you want more than status quo, if you really want to transform your life after kids, you must treat the cause and not the symptoms. In the health and wellness space, we use this phrase all the time. For example, if you have constant bloating and stomach pain after eating due to a food allergy, you can take antacids or digestive enzymes to stop the bloat and pain (the symptom), but until you remove the food that you're allergic to (the cause), you'll never be as healthy as you could be; what's more, the overuse of antacids/enzymes could have side effects that create other symptoms you don't want.

In the same way, if you focus your entire being on your kids' lives to feel better about this phase of life (symptom), you'll never be as fulfilled as you want to be unless you focus on your own purpose and passions for life (cause). Plus, you could end up experiencing the unwanted side effect of pushing your kids away or putting stress on their relationships.

I can tell you from experience that finding purpose and having something that lights me up and gets me excited to wake up in the morning outside of my kids saved me. I am not being my typical dramatic self when I say this, and that does not make me any less of a mom. I happen to adore my kids. But building the Life after Kids brand and business with Dr. Lynne has filled my heart and grown me in ways that I could never have imagined. It's made me a happier person and it's made me a better mom. Without a doubt, it's softened the blow of my kids growing up and leaving home because, rather than constantly lamenting what was, I have so much reason to look forward to what will be.

In finding my purpose, I found myself again. I'm a mom and I always will be, but I'm also Brooke Stillwell, a vibrant woman excited about her life and what her future holds. And if I can get there, so can you. So, I'll ask you, what is it you want to do now? What sets your heart on fire? Are there causes you are passionate about? Was there a skill you acquired prior to kids that you'd like to revisit or something new you'd like to learn? Maybe you want a new career. Perhaps you want to start a job, take a class, pick up a hobby, travel, or volunteer. As my husband likes to remind me from time to time, "The best thing you have going for you now is that you can do anything you want to do, and the hardest thing you have to deal with is that you can do anything you want to do!"

You may feel a little overwhelmed, and that's completely normal. You have a lot to think about and a whole new purpose to build! But don't worry we're here to help. You've already taken the first step. The rest is a series of taking the next right steps to get you where you want to go.

Chapter 2

What Do I Do Now?

By Dr. Lynne

Building the Foundation

Before we can reveal the steps for finding more purpose, elevating your health and relationships, and generally soaring in your Life after Kids, you'll need to do a little groundwork. If you're like so many of our readers, you're just emerging on the other side of a long season of motherhood, and you've been laser focused on the needs and wants of the humans you've been raising for the last 18+ years.

Can we just take a moment to celebrate that achievement? You've borne children either from your body or from your heart, and you've stood by them every day, kissing their bruises and sharing all of their wins and disappointments. It's been a thankless job at times. It's been harder than anyone could have prepared you for, but I'm betting you'd also agree that it's been far more worthwhile than anything else you've ever done or could imagine. At the end of the day, you've likely sacrificed so much for your children.

If you're like most moms, there hasn't been a whole lot of time or energy left over to spend on yourself.

Ironically, this is exactly where you will find much of the beauty and the opportunities available to you at this time in your life. Suddenly, your whole life is ahead of you again. The good news is there's some more time left over now to focus on your own personal happiness and fulfillment. The bad news—it's not just more time that will guarantee your success.

Trust me when I tell you that you will benefit so much from having a solid inner foundation that will reinforce you and steer you toward what you need the most from here forward. I also want to help you determine what you *don't* need and what's not serving you right now. The cornerstone piece of this foundation is to know yourself better as a woman who still has so much life to live ahead of her. I hope you agree with me this is the very best place to start your journey.

All women has their own unique combination of factors that together have the potential to synergistically produce their happiest and most fulfilled life. In this chapter, we'll show you some tools and exercises to help you tease out your very own personal combination, setting you up for your best life. While we can't tell you exactly what that magical combination is for you, we certainly can tell what will likely *not* get you there.

You Won't Get There With Mo' Money

Recently, the results of an 85-year Harvard study that studied well-being were released.[1] One of the major conclusions of this study was this: Beyond a certain income threshold, researchers determined that adding more wealth will not significantly increase your happiness. This landmark study is especially remarkable because it's one of the longest running and most diverse studies ever conducted on this topic.

As far as the pursuit of happiness by accumulating more wealth goes, if you're struggling to pay your bills and have little to none left over, then increasing your income will in fact increase overall happiness, according to the Harvard researchers.[1] Within the Life after Kids community we like to refer to this milestone as "graduating from survival mode." However, if you're reasonably secure financially and generally able to meet your basic needs like food and shelter, for instance, additional expendable income will *not* make you feel or be happier. In fact it could do just the opposite.

Of course, more money can arguably give you better access and provide more potentially life-enriching experiences. However, when it comes to your innermost state of emotional health and wellness, the researchers proved that money won't significantly improve your inner well-being. If you're feeling miserable or lost in this phase of life, you'll likely continue to feel miserable or lost, only with more expendable income. Or worse, you might become even *more distressed* than before because your conclusion that money would fix your problems won't prove to be true.

This brings back memories of dancing my butt off in the club with my friends in the '90s singing "It's like the more money we come across, the more problems we see" at the top of our lungs. Ha! Biggie Smalls had it right all along.

You Won't Get There Through Your Kids

Brace yourself because this may sting just a bit. If your dream is to have a close relationship with your grown kids and they are your *only* outlet to direct your energy into, it's highly probable this could backfire on you. For one, if your kids are well adjusted and have lives of their own, they're going to want, hope, and expect you to have the same. You might think there's some value in being a martyr when it comes to them, but too much mothering can and will most likely smother your children. I've also known moms who remain at their older kids' beck and call only to complain they still don't get to see their kids or grandkids as much as they'd like.

Your kids will respect you more if you have a healthy balance between prioritizing their needs and prioritizing your own needs. They will not only respect you more, but the law of attraction also dictates they'll be more likely to be drawn to spend time with you if you have your own purpose and reasons for living outside of them. If you give of yourself and your time with the expectation that they now should return the favor, just know you might run the risk of pushing them away.

You Won't Get There with More Fun and Games

As amazing as sitting on a tropical beach drinking champagne and reading a good book sounds, if you did that day in and day out for weeks on end, you'd end up pretty bored wouldn't you? Too often, women seek to fill their days with as many "fun" activities they can possibly muster. Their schedule is chock-full of lunch dates, pickleball games, and tailgates. As I write this, I'm smiling because even I can admit that actually sounds pretty great. But c'mon, only for a couple of months or so, right? If you approach your life after kids this way, many of you would likely discover an inconvenient truth.

If all work and no play makes Jack a dull boy, then all play and no work makes Jill an unfulfilled and restless camper. Let me explain. When your kids are grown, you typically appreciate the times your family is all together under one roof more, and you become acutely aware that these moments are fleeting. You can also more fully lean into the appreciation of each day you're given more and more as you navigate the more frequent losses and illnesses of your peers and loved ones as you age. It's this juxtaposition that helps us feel more deeply and encourages us to be more grateful for what we have while we have it.

It works the same when it comes to having fun. In relative terms, something is fun *because* we don't get to do it every day. The activity is, by its nature, fun because it contrasts with the mundane. Therefore, the more often you repeat something that started as fun, the less fun and the more mundane it becomes. If your only goal is to have fun, it won't be easy to do. You'll have to keep amping up your efforts to prevent your fun activities from becoming as repetitive as your regular day-to-day undertakings.

I recently heard about the Buddhist concept of a hungry ghost. As the term goes, hungry ghosts are beings who are tormented by desires that can never be satiated or filled. According to these teachings, they're destined to wander the land, continually eating or drinking, for example, but never feeling full. In people, they show up as our insatiable and often misplaced desires.

Some of you may find yourself always chasing more fun in your empty nest, with it never seeming to be enough. This is your hungry ghost.

You Won't Get There through Outside Validation

Back in the day, I was a dedicated trumpet player. Making music is one of the things I've rediscovered in later life that provides me with a true sense of joy. I started playing in fifth grade with the other middle schoolers whose parents had signed them up to try an instrument and join the band. I'd been taking piano lessons for about five years, so I had a jumpstart on reading music and seemed to learn faster than most of my new bandmates. I'm the youngest of two girls—the little sister—forever trailing behind my cool and sporty older sister. Suddenly, I was good at something, too! It was a heady feeling. My teacher, Mrs. Chisholm singled me out for playing so well in front of the whole class. That validation felt so amazing that the chance of earning more made me want to go home and practice every day for hours.

Looking back, I feel so bad for my parents having to endure the merciless honking and squeaking that regularly poured out of my room. If you're the mom of a child who's attempted to learn a new instrument, then you, too, have likely endured this remarkable form of eardrum torture, and I salute you.

In eighth grade, I was promoted to the high school band. From there, I auditioned and earned a place in an exclusive ensemble made up of all of the best music students in the city. Each of the novel achievements I accumulated felt good, but I found myself looking for recognition and validation from my new band teacher, Dr. Smith. I missed the regular stroking of my ego from Mrs. Chisholm.

Unfortunately, Dr. Smith wasn't into giving much positive feedback, and he could be harsh and critical at times. I quickly became anxious and lost confidence in myself and my abilities. For a while, I worked harder. No matter what I did, I never seemed to be able to elicit the recognition from Dr. Smith that I was craving. Instead of being confident in my abilities with a solid sense of belief in myself, I had learned to listen to the feedback from others as evidence of my worth. I had conditioned myself to place more value in others' opinions of me than I did my own opinions of myself.

This still feels raw as I share it with you. It's something I'm vigilant of to this day. I share this because I want you to check in with your motivations as well. Are you doing certain things for the validation you might gain from someone in your life even if those things aren't bringing you joy or aren't right for you? Do you care more than you should about how others see you or what they think of you? Maybe you don't see any harm in that.

For someone who's conditioned to thrive on outside validation, compliments can be compared to that initial flush-faced feeling you get when you take your first few sips of a delicious cocktail, and any vocal feedback that's negative can be devastating. If you're blind to this part of your personality, you might find yourself on that hamster wheel again doing whatever you can to get outside approval. Once you acknowledge the extent to which you seek approval from others to justify your worth, you'll need to stay on guard and check in often to make sure you're doing things you truly love and enjoy and not from the urge to appease the critics in your life. It's another kind of hungry ghost. There can never be enough compliments or admiration from the outside to fill you up.

The greatest satisfaction to be had is when your foremost validation comes from within.

What Exactly Do We Need in Our Life after Kids?

Now that we've established some common ways to get derailed in this phase of life, let's direct our attention to what's most likely to bring you closer to your best life after raising your kids. As I've observed in my own life, I tend to feel the happiest and most at peace during the times when my basic needs are getting met, and I'd venture to guess it's the same for you. I found it so helpful when I first realized this and subsequently started to tune in to my primary needs several years ago.

Remember when your babies were little? I can't believe I'm going to say this, but in some ways things were so easy back then. When they cried, only a few things could be wrong. Either you had to feed them, burp them, change them, or rock them to sleep. Years later, I only wish my teenager and my 30-something son came with such a short list of grievances to decode. Fortunately, when it comes to our basic needs as midlife women, the list is shorter than you might think.

You'll Need Your Health

The idea of the basic needs of humans comes from psychologist Abraham Maslow, who described our earthly needs as a pyramid with each increasing level becoming more complex and more connected to our purest sense of self. Maslow felt that we must meet our basic primal needs, such as food, water, and shelter before we can move up the ladder to work on getting our other requirements. You can't skip a level. Like in the game of Ms. Pac-Man, you've got to eat up all of the pellets to finish the level before you can move on to the next.

Many women in our community are truly struggling, financially and/or emotionally. They're trying to keep their heads above water, living in survival mode, day in and day out. It can be a scary and frustrating place to be, especially if no matter what you do you feel as if you're taking one step ahead and two steps back. Survival mode is when you're using all of your time and energy to put out fires and maintain the status quo leaving no time to work on yourself, improve your health, or save for a rainy day. For your sake, Dr. Brooke and I are hoping you are reading this ready and able to devote time, energy, and focus on your future—we're going to be so much more effective for you if you've managed to square away your basic day-to-day survival.

Even if you are stable emotionally and financially, many of you are presented with some alarming physical symptoms at this stage in your life. This commonly stems from a combination of factors, including hormonal imbalances and menopause, undiagnosed food intolerances, consuming too many processed foods or not enough exercise combined with living a habitually stressed life. These health challenges can land you squarely back in survival mode, zapping your energy and leaving little time for much else than tending to your health. Although diagnosing and finding answers to any individualized health problems is outside of the scope of this book, we will give you some practical and foundational advice Chapter 6 to apply if you are indeed struggling with your health. For those who are health challenged right now, finish this chapter and then feel free to skip to Chapter 6 before returning back to pick up where you left off.

You'll Need a Village

You're going to need a few more things beyond your basic survival needs. The next level up in your needs pyramid is to allocate energy to meet your need for love and belonging. For many women, life will feel lonelier now. Our houses are quieter. We're missing the connections we had with our kids and, in many cases, the connections with the parents of our kids' friends. Most of us understand the difference between surface-level type relationships and high-quality, give-and-take relationships with true companions who help us feel seen and heard. Most women in our community say they are craving more of the latter yet find themselves struggling to develop these types of friendships.

Finding like-minded women (or men) to share your highs and lows of this season can make all the difference in feeling happy and fulfilled. It's such an important topic that it will be the primary focus of Chapters 8 and 9. If you have a spouse or partner, refreshing and strengthening your bond as a couple becomes that much more important now that you're empty-nesting. According to the Mayo Clinic,[2] we're happier, less stressed, and better able to deal with difficult times when we have a solid support system. The results of that same long-running Harvard research study from the start of this chapter goes as far as to prove that the most important and tell-tale predictor of human happiness, life satisfaction, and well-being is the quality of our relationships.

You might be a very reserved individual, fed up with people in general or dissatisfied with the friendships you've made along the way. However, you feel about the current state of your relationships, the science clearly shows there are abundant emotional and physical advantages for those who have people in their lives whom they can rely upon. It's important to know that as a human being you're hardwired as a social creature. You need others and they need you, especially now.

You'll Need To Love Yourself

Has there been a time you've been seated across from your child, and in that moment, you felt an overwhelming sense of pride and gratitude? Not because of their achievements or how they look on the outside but simply because of their very existence and what that means to you as their mom? If you answered yes, the time has come for you, sweet mama, to direct that same intensity of love and appreciation toward yourself.

This is a huge part of the next level of your happiness and fulfillment. In addition to the joy that you experience from your grown children, you can create within yourself a self-sustaining love of who you are fundamentally as a woman. Happiness and fulfillment comes from cultivating the belief that your unique make-up of talents, personality, and character, given the opportunity, can make the world a better place.

If the last paragraph makes you cringe or squirm a little, you're not alone. When it comes to talking about ourselves, it seems that, for most moms, it's our least favorite topic. You may even feel that it's selfish or vain to do so.

Answer this: Are you willing to admit that there are traits or talents that you don't like or would like to change about yourself? I'll venture to bet most would answer yes to that question. Why is it so easy to spot where we lack or fall short and harder to see what makes us remarkable? One of my favorite quotes by Tony Robbins is, "What's wrong is always available, but so is what's right." If this is true and you're easily able to spot when you fall short or where you're lacking, then it stands to reason that you could also train yourself to notice what's good and right about you, where you shine and stand out in the best way.

For some of you, it will in fact take actual *training*. Learning to look at the bright side or in this case the "right side" takes practice. However, pivoting your thoughts to focus on the positive is a powerful tool to employ in those times that you're wallowing in the past or feeling irrelevant or invisible now that your kids are grown. We call this concept "reframing." Reframing is the practice of switching a negative or disempowering thought into a positive, irrefutable fact. For example, thinking "My house feels so quiet and empty now that my kids are gone. I don't know what to do with myself." becomes "This is a new chapter of my life, and I have more freedom to focus on my passions and personal growth. I have more time to explore new hobbies and experiences that can enrich my life and create new memories."

You'll probably falter until you build this new "muscle" with enough repetition until it becomes commonplace to think first about what is good about your situation before evaluating it for the downsides. Take heart, and keep trying. Choosing to exercise the power of reframing your thoughts is a game changer.

You'll Need a Sense of Purpose

If you manage to successfully meet all of the previous needs described, you'll be sitting in rare air. And there's still one more tier to climb. The cherry on top, the pinnacle of the pyramid, is this: As a women and mother, you have a compelling need to live with a sense of purpose. Your purpose is the practical expression of who you are and what you do best. Simply put, it's something that has the power to propel you out of your bed each morning because you're compelled to go and do it. Your purpose helps you to feel more alive, and it validates your uniqueness.

If this concept is new to you, it might be helpful to examine some common symptoms that present when women, like us moms with grown kids, are lacking a sense of purpose. Do you experience a certain level of anxiety without reason? Do you feel like you lack motivation or direction? Losing joy in your activities is common, and in the worst cases, this can leave you feeling numb to what's happening around you. You might find yourself dreaming less, shrinking your hopes for your life, or thinking "What's the point?" When someone is lacking purpose for a long time, it can even manifest as physical symptoms or poor health.

Your purpose is the very reason for which you exist. It's easy to see how being a mom fits that bill. It was probably the major driving force for each of your days until now. It is and likely always will be a central purpose for your life, but your mom work has slowed, and you've been designated as a seasonal worker. How can you find more purpose to fill your life with meaning again?

I want to point out that in some cases you don't find your purpose; it finds you. I'm Christian, so I believe God has designed a plan for us with our purpose in mind. If you are not a Christian, feel free to chalk it up to the universe, luck, karma, or whatever matches your personal beliefs. Sometimes, we stumble into something so well suited for us that fits our unique talents and sparks joy for us, but it isn't convenient, practical, or even logical. Take for example my friend, Char, who is funny, kind and usually the best dressed women in the room. Char moved to Puerto Rico a few years back with her husband, leaving their grown kids back in the mainland United States.

As Char was assimilating in her new surroundings, she kept encountering stray dogs everywhere she went. After Hurricane Maria devastated Puerto Rico, thousands of abandoned dogs formed wild packs to survive. Char became acquainted with some women and men who spent their days rescuing these dogs. These helpless creatures are often found starving to death and dehydrated, suffering from human mistreatment and living in deplorable conditions. She eventually started a nonprofit, UpShot Dog Rescue, and in just a few years, she's saved hundreds of dogs' lives through fostering and adoption to loving and stable homes where they can be showered with they love and attention they deserve.

It's remarkable because her work involves tenuous adventures in ditches, culverts, and abandoned warehouses of San Juan to uncover these sweet souls in need. She's often found hands deep in the filth, poop, and disease of these vulnerable creatures, yet with her polished appearance and wide smile you'd never guess it. It's not entirely logical, but her level of commitment to saving these pups is inspiring, and the personal risks she takes to save them are seriously impressive. I'm so thankful that Char's purpose found her for two reasons: I care deeply about the protection of defenseless animals and I sleep better at night knowing there are women with this level of gumption, like Char, in the world. And secondly, I simply couldn't imagine life without our sweet Puerto Rican *sato*, Journey, who thanks us every day in her own way, either with a prolonged snuggle or a knowing tail wag.

It's normal to have more than one purpose in a lifetime, and it's entirely normal to have more than one purpose at one time. I want to make it clear that your purpose doesn't have to be your job or just what you do. Some of you have amazing careers that captivate you and give you a purposeful feeling each day even though there might be many aspects of your job that you actually dislike. This amount of purpose might be enough for you, but if you're having some of those symptoms we mentioned above, you could consider adding, creating, or developing something else to bring you more purpose.

For those who do work that would be characterized as less meaningful or lacking purpose, we hope you'll become inspired to find something on the side, separate from your work designed to bring more purpose to your life. For example, a mom friend of mine teaches yoga and Pilates classes for her kids and their moms on the weekends. She does have a nine-to-five, but it doesn't revolve around fitness and mindfulness, which have become her deepest passions as she's gotten older. She doesn't charge much, and it's so fun attending her classes. It's clear she loves her work, and she imparts some knowledge of the body to all who attend her classes—everyone wins.

As I mentioned, purpose doesn't have to be only what you do. It can be intertwined with *who* you are. And it doesn't have to be big. Maybe you don't feel compelled to save orphans or start a nonprofit. Maybe you're wondering if you can find purpose without having to change your life much at all. You absolutely can, and I have the perfect example! There's a man, named Ron, at my local grocery store who works behind the customer service desk. Everyone in my community knows him; Ron is basically a celebrity in my town. He has a remarkably quiet and gentle spirit and is great with any and all tasks you throw at him, but it's actually his smile that stands out and is the reason he's so well known. You have to smile back at Ron, and at the risk of sounding dramatic, I simply feel a little bit better about the world immediately after spending time in his presence.

It feels as if Ron's main purpose is to bring a smile to everyone he meets. And notably, he achieves his purpose in part by just being himself and doing his work with excellence. It isn't necessarily monumental or groundbreaking. Or is it? He works with roughly 50–100 people a day. If he leaves each person feeling better than before, imagine that ripple effect! I can think of no more deserving person and almost no one who is more fueled by an important purpose than Ron.

Ron is just one example. Here's a question to think deeper: Why do you exist right now at this very moment? Are you meant to be a leader in your social network, to inspire others to achieve big things, or to thrive on your journey and impart life's lessons along your way? Are you meant to bring kindness to others, to give encouragement where it's needed or to simply bring a smile to everyone you come across? Raising a family and setting a positive example for your children is a significant path to purpose. After doing that for so many years, how can you now reach outside of your core family and find more purpose doing something that you enjoy for years to come?

A few years ago, I came up with a formula for finding more purpose. If you're a visual learner, I think it will help.

Your Unique Abilities + Passion × Urgent Need = Your Purpose

Your purpose is the combination of your unique abilities added to something you feel passionate about multiplied by a pressing or urgent need in your community or the world. The greater the need and alignment with your talents and passions, the greater the return on your time, focus, and energy in providing you with more purpose and life satisfaction. My buddy Ron has his unique abilities on display, and he has combined that with his sincere passion to help others feel more positive and at ease. In what areas do you feel passionate?

These ingredients coming together can result in a beautiful synergy that becomes exponentially larger wherever there is an urgent demand. Char found a pressing need in the mounting homeless dog population in Puerto Rico. Is there something that you feel compelled to fix or do based on a glaring need in your community or the world? Perhaps there's a family in your neighborhood who needs your help urgently. The world will always need you and your unique abilities. For someone or something, *you* are the answer. Symbiotically, those needs can provide you with more of the meaning and purpose that you're lacking right now.

As I alluded earlier, sometimes your purpose just falls into your lap, and sometimes you really have to go searching for it. If you're in the second boat, there are five helpful clues from Don Clifton's book *Now, Discover Your Strengths*[3] that can lead you to your unique talents and gifts. When you are naturally good at something, it usually brings an immense amount of energy, joy, and satisfaction. A great place to start to look for more purpose is to start where you are naturally gifted. These clues can be used as green flags to discern whether an activity, vocation, or cause will be well-matched to your natural talents in addition to bringing you a new sense of purpose.

Yearning

A yearning or desire to do more of something is a strong clue in finding purpose. When you find yourself drawn to an activity, organization, or creative task, take notice. What might start out as a strong yearning to do something creative, for instance, could morph into a business making beautiful art. Or perhaps you just want to use your time and talents to bring comfort to others so you make blankets or mix essential oils with lotions to give to sick kids or seniors. Maybe it's not creative pursuits you yearn for but intellectual pursuits instead. You could engage a natural yearning to teach or help friends strategize in your area of expertise.

Satisfaction

If yearning is what we feel before we engage in an activity of purpose, satisfaction is what we feel after we are finished doing it. Gauge your level of satisfaction as a very strong clue that an activity or role is purposeful for you. If volunteer work is very satisfying for you, this is a great way to find purpose. Maybe you miss cooking for your family because the feeling of satisfaction in making delicious food is satisfying. In that case, you could dedicate yourself to bringing food or baking treats to those people in your life celebrating birthdays for a year, or you could cook for a widow in your circle or a family experiencing a sickness or loss.

Rapid Learning

Being a quick learner is a sign your aptitude for that task or project is above average. What can you learn that will make a difference for you or others? I have a friend in her fifties who taught herself digital marketing starting at ground zero. Before she got started, she could barely log into Facebook. Now she does freelance work and helps local brick-and-mortar businesses advertise their services in their communities. She's paid well, and her new line of work gives her a sense of purpose. Maybe you're a whiz at learning languages. You could start a club with friends or help new citizens learn the language.

Glimpses of Excellence

Your path to purpose is lit by small glimpses of excellence along the way. One of my best friends is an amazing doctor and clinician. Her patients love her in part because she has a way of explaining things in a powerful way that really motivates people to change their behavior. You could say she is an excellent communicator. As she transitions out of her full-time clinician role, she is finding purpose in developing videos and courses for teens, communicating ways to adopt a healthier mindset.

Flow State

Have you ever been so lost in something you were doing that time almost seemed to stand still? When you looked at the clock, you could hardly believe so much time had passed. Some people call this being *in the zone*. This flow state is another important clue to those pursuits that have the most potential to bring you more purpose.

One Clear Path to Purpose

I'm going to level with you. Despite my extensive work and personal experience with helping women find more purpose, at times it's still a tricky thing to uncover. In part because no one else will ever know *you* as well as you know yourself. That is exactly where we can help.

In the next chapter I'll share some of the practical ways I came to know myself better. Knowing myself better has led me to more fully accept myself for who I am, how I'm wired, and what I do best. Fully accepting myself has led to me loving myself enough to have the discipline and confidence to pursue the things that bring me the greatest joy and satisfaction. Pursuing the things that I love has led me to take more chances, learn new lessons, and grow more as a person. Taking chances, learning lessons, and growing as a person has led me to the greater realization that fulfillment in life comes from finding a vehicle to bring value to others in the special way that only I can do. That brings us full circle, doesn't it?

In my experience, this same path is the way for every mom to find more purpose after raising children. *Your purpose is your vehicle for bringing value to others in the unique way that only you can do.* For Dr. Brooke and I, along with so many of the women in our Life after Kids community, it begins with getting to know yourself better. As Julie Andrews sang in my favorite movie of all time, *The Sound of Music*, starting at the very beginning "is the very best place to start." So, buckle up, mama—let's continue our journey together and help you find your way.

Chapter 3

Finding Your Way

By Dr. Lynne

A New Perspective

When I was about two years old, my older sister first noticed my right eye was turning cross-eyed while we were playing together one afternoon. As the story goes, she tried for weeks to tell my Mom that something was wrong with my eye, but she wasn't able to convince my mom to take much notice or action.

Let's take a moment in reverence for the moms from the '70s and '80s, shall we? In general, they were pretty hardcore. I admire how little they worried and especially how little they had to worry about. Picture how differently it must have been to be a mom then compared to today. No seatbelt for every child . . . who needs seat belts anyway? Your kid falls down . . . as long as nothing's broken, you're good! Get up, brush it off! No cell phones and zero idea where your children go once they leave your house? No worries! They know to just head home when the street lights come on.

In any case, as it turns out, there was in fact something wrong with my eye. It took my mom seeing for herself the way my right eye lazily turned inward while I was focused on staying inside the lines in my coloring book one afternoon. From that moment, it was a matter of days until my two-year-old little body was plopped in Dr. Lawton's huge, padded chair. Lawton, the optometrist, expertly switched out different lenses for me to look through and asked me questions as I stared at symbols. How challenging must it be to determine prescription for glasses for a child not yet old enough to read the letters on the eye chart?

I still have my first pair of eyeglasses that were prescribed that day. The lenses are almost two inches thick and they're only 4 inches wide, just big enough to fit my tiny head. The long curved temple-tips scooped well under my ear, pointing forward to my jaw, designed that way so they would stay put on the head of a toddler who doesn't understand she should keep them on at all times.

If you've had the experience of getting a new pair of prescription glasses, you know what happens next. When you first slip them on, your whole world comes into focus suddenly. Everything seems a little sharper and closer—your perspective shifts. It's feels as if everything around you changes in an instant.

Seeing Clearly: The Four Ds

Learning new things about your authentic self and why you do the things you do has a similar effect. For most of your adult life, you've been their mom. When your kids grow up and leave, it's as if you have to find yourself and who you are all over again.

As you make new connections and develop insights about yourself, suddenly the way you see yourself changes. When you change the way you see yourself, you create a ripple effect. In the same way that eyeglasses are a tool to help you see more clearly, Dr. Brooke and I believe you need to clarify four major areas to reconnect and know yourself better. We call them the Four Ds: (1) Determine your non-negotiables; (2) Develop a compelling plan for your future; (3) Discover where you shine; and finally (4) Dismantle your blind spots. We will give you some ways to dig into each one so you can relearn who you are now and sharpen your focus on what you want in this next chapter.

Determine Your Non-Negotiables

One of my favorite things to do on a weekday afternoon alone is to browse the aisles at Whole Foods. I'll grab a cart, head to the cafe to order a steaming hot Golden Milk Latte, and spend a couple of hours indulging my senses and feeling so good about the healthy food I'll be bringing home to my family.

If you've shopped at a Whole Foods, too, you get that it's typically a more fun, attractive, and nurturing experience than those had at other grocery stores. My husband and I have even started a few date nights there!

Companies like Whole Foods don't leave their success to chance. They adopt a specific set of core values that guides them in making all of their important business decisions, from the colors they use in an end cap display to whom they choose to partner with. If I were to tell you just a few of Whole Foods' core values—for example "We sell the highest quality natural and organic foods" or "We satisfy and delight our customers"—you might even recognize the Whole Foods brand by those statements alone.

How can this customary business strategy possibly apply to your life? You may not realize it, but every single decision you make from the clothes you put on each morning to the people you spend your time with to the places where you spend your hard-earned dollars is a direct indication of *your* own core values.

Every human's actions and behaviors are dictated from their own individual set of values. The biggest difference among us is that some people are consciously aware of the values that guide them while many others act without any awareness of the values behind the decisions they make. The greatest downside in the second method is you're much more likely to succumb to your momentary emotional whims, possibly foregoing your long-term happiness in favor of your short-term comfort.

Here are three crucial ways that, determining your personal values, can bolster you during this major life transition:

1. When you consider first what matters most, you will simply make better decisions. Instead of deciding on an impulse what career path you should take or where you should move after your kids leave home, filtering those decisions through your personal set of values will help you make more right moves and less wrong ones for your future.

2. Clarifying your values will reduce overwhelm. Overwhelm is the number one reason we stay stagnant in life circumstances that are less than we hoped for. When you're clear on your personal values, you can more quickly and easily discard the options that would drive you away from what is most important to you. This leads to fewer choices and less overwhelm overall.

3. Finally, getting clear on your values helps you be more resilient amidst life's setbacks. When a relationship dwindles or other challenging life changes like a job loss or divorce occurs, a mismatch of values is often to blame. By correctly placing the blame on the circumstances, we have a greater chance of keeping our integrity and self-assuredness amidst life's storms. To paraphrase a friend and mentor Dr. Pat Gentempo, when you contradict your values, it leads to consequences that are a direct reflection of how considerable that difference is. In other words, the bigger the gap between your value and the choices you make, the more likely you are to suffer pain, regret, and difficulties in life.

Exercise: Identifying Your Core Values

In our Life after Kids community, we help women determine their personal core values using the following exercise. Ideally, you'll come out of this exercise with a set of words or short statements that perfectly communicates who you are as a person and what you truly hold most dear. Throughout your life, it's entirely possible that your values will change, especially following life transitions. That's precisely why this exercise is so timely right now. It's unlikely that what you valued most in your pre-family 20s is the same as what you value now in your post child-rearing midlife.

Go to www.lifeafterkids.com/book to print the list of core value prompts that we've curated just for you. Here are a few questions to get you started thinking about what you care most about. Is health a value that you want to commit to in your life in this next phase? How about determination, forgiveness, courage, or faith? What is a brand you are loyal to and why? We often shop and buy products from companies that share our values.

Here are a few more helpful questions to consider before completing this exercise:

- How do you prefer to spend the bulk of your time?
- What do you spend your money on outside of your necessities?
- What topics do you tend to discuss with others over and over?
- In what areas of your life do you often take action to improve?
- In what areas of your life have you successfully set and accomplished long-term goals?

Read the word list carefully and circle the words that you feel at least *50%* sure could belong on your final draft of values. After you've picked this initial word set, you will conduct a tournament to cut down to your final 5–10 values. To do this, go through your initial list and give each word either an A or a B grade. The A grade words are those words that strongly resonate with you. If you have trouble deciding, refer back to the starter questions for some direction. *Pro tip: if you're on the fence with a particular word, it's a B.*

Next, print the tournament bracket from the download and write your words in A–B pairs on the tournament diagram for the first round. It's perfectly fine to have more B words than A words at this point. In that case, pick a winner from all of the A–B match-ups; following that, you will rematch the winning words with the remaining unpaired B words. Continue choosing winners for each pair and move the winners on to the next round to compete against the other winners. Continue until you have your top core value. The final 5–9 competing words of the tournament will become your list of your own core values.

If you've completed this exercise, congratulations! You now have a list of personal core values to guide you. You can keep them as a word list or you could go one step further and build statements from those single words. Dr. Brooke and I recently completed a similar exercise and here's our list of Life after Kids core values with corresponding statements that guides us in this important work.

- Community: Every woman deserves to feel seen, valued, and supported beyond motherhood.
- Distinction: A personal approach, combined with the elements of surprise and fun, sparks joy and loyalty.
- Celebration: Celebrating women as they navigate their personal journey back to self.
- Guidance: Guiding women to holistically recognize their own strengths to create a life they love after kids.
- Impact: Women create the most positive impact for themselves and others by realizing their worth and using their talents to make a difference.

Whatever you stand for, putting those values into words or statements will allow you to effectively keep your priorities clear and future decisions easier. When you're faced with a difficult decision, turn first to your core values for the best answer to keep you on the right trajectory toward your best life.

Develop a Compelling Plan For Your Future

"By failing to prepare, you are preparing to fail"
—*Ben Franklin*

The next stop on your way back to your authentic self is to create a vision for your future and a solid plan to get there.

A few years ago, my sister and I re-discovered jigsaw puzzles. We were together with our families in Florida during two of the rainiest weeks of that summer. We had to find things to do besides drinking wine and watching the raindrops as they incessantly rolled down the window panes. When we came across a 1,000-piece puzzle left behind by previous renters, we dove in excitedly, methodically separating the corner pieces from the middle pieces.

We talked, laughed, and shared old memories as we puzzled each morning and night. In just a few days, we'd reconnected as sisters and friends, felt accomplished in having completed a challenging puzzle, and best of all, we discovered a new hobby together that we continue to enjoy.

Would you even think of putting a jigsaw puzzle together without the picture on the box top to guide you? Technically, it can be done. It sure makes puzzling more difficult though, doesn't it? It's hard to create something you can't see clearly. Armed with a clear picture and a plan, it's true there's still no guarantee of success. However, *without* a plan, statistically you have a much greater chance of failure. With a good plan and the right action, the odds of success are heavily weighted in your favor.

In rediscovering who you are, you also get to decide *what* you want. There is so much opportunity ahead, but you're more likely to dwell in the past and mourn what you've lost when there's no exciting or compelling vision for what IS possible for your future.

Exercise: Completing Your Goals Framework

Dr. Brooke and I designed the *Life after Kids Goals Framework* to keep your vision and plan for your future, easy to do, fun, and highly relevant to this phase of life. Listen, we know that setting goals can be kind of scary. The thought of taking pen to paper and writing something you want for your life carries a large risk, doesn't it? We tend not to like disappointing others and we *really* dislike disappointing ourselves. We're going to ask you to take a leap of faith here, and despite the risk of failure that comes with setting goals, we're going to ask you to do it anyway.

Go to www.lifeafterkids/book to get your copy of the Life after Kids Goals Framework. We've identified the eight most relevant categories for moms to create a vision and plan for their lives. If you're new to goal-setting, we recommend starting small and picking a few easily attainable goals in each of the categories. It's perfectly okay to cherry-pick a few goals to get started and to help you feel successful in this process. When you make early wins, it propels you to keep going and from there it's more likely to become a sustainable habit. Congratulate yourself each time and celebrate in a meaningful way when you do something you set out to do. Then use that positive momentum to spur on even more action.

Our recommendation when doing self-reflection exercises like these is to find an inspiring setting outside of your everyday four walls. Go somewhere new and creatively stimulating, for instance a garden that grounds you or a coffee shop where you can both vibe on the caffeinated energy and get lost in your thoughts. I've personally found it next to impossible to achieve this type of heart-driven clarity when I sit down in my own home, knowing that my dishes and laundry are waiting or that someone could yell "Mom, I need you!" at any minute. You do you, girl, but my bet is that you'll figure out exactly what I mean if you try to do this exercise from the same sofa where you watch Netflix every night.

Our second piece of advice is to be prepared to feel awkward and clunky at first, especially if this is your first time doing an exercise like this. You may even hear a voice that says "This is too hard" or "I feel dumb" when getting started. To this we say, *do it anyway*. Anything worth doing is usually hard, clunky, awkward, or all three at once! We promise, it gets easier, and it will be so worthwhile when you put the work in. Even if you just learn one small new thing about yourself or come up with just one important goal, that little change could be an important catalyst for a transformation you've been craving.

To have something you've never had, you're going to have to do something you've never done. As we say to our members of the Life after Kids membership community, you're not growing *until* it feels unnatural and uncomfortable. When you step out on a limb far enough to feel the stretch, you're usually onto something good.

Exercise: Casting Your Life Vision

What do you ultimately want for your life? What do you envision when you feel the most encouraged for the years yet to come? Dream big! Go ahead, give yourself permission to send your mind to places that you might not think possible, but for which your heart desires.

Once you've brainstormed the big picture, let's narrow the focus to just the next 12 months. What is your life vision for the next year? List all the things that you want to see, do, and accomplish. In general, we overestimate what we can do in a day and we drastically underestimate what we can do in a year. A convincing plan can help take you to places you've so far only dreamed of going.

Next, pick the top three things you consider to be the most important goals for you to reach in the next year. Consider your newly cemented values to ensure these goals are in sync with what you've defined as your highest priorities. For example, if you'd like to finish your degree but you know being free to come and go is a personal value right now, you could decide to do something else or find a solution that accomplishes both, such as enrolling exclusively in online schooling.

Now, establish your *why*. Why are these goals important to you? How would your life be different if you were to accomplish them? More powerful even—ask yourself what your life would be like if you don't do what you say is important? List all the ways, big and small. Keep this list at the ready. I use my notes app on my iPhone. When the going gets tough or you're feeling unmotivated, refer back to all of the reasons you began this journey in the first place so you can dig deeper and keep going.

Finally, identify at least *one* thing to act on in the next 90 days to reach your desired goal. List your action step(s) to your goal and hold yourself accountable to BIG action in the next quarter.

Look at you go! If you've followed our lead, you now have an exciting plan for the next year and you've thought deeply about what you really want for your future beyond that. This is more than half the battle, and it will completely separate you from your peers in a good way. Your circumstances could change and things may shift a little, but executing on a compelling plan that allows you to continue growing in multiple areas of your life and also refocuses you on what you want and need most is a true success in itself.

Discover Where You Shine

I've come to learn through my work as a Strengths coach that every person on earth does at least one thing expertly. The tragic part is most people, moms included, are not aware of the very things they do best and how those things make them truly one-of-a-kind. Part of the reason is when you're really good at something, it generally comes so easy and automatic to you that you completely take it for granted *because* of the very fact that it does come so naturally to you.

Taking it one harmful step further—some women unwittingly *project* their gifts onto their loved ones, meaning because it's so effortless for them, they assume and expect others (usually their kids or spouse) to perform as well or better in the same areas and they become easily disappointed or critical when they do not. They have totally overlooked that only they possess those talents and others have alternate ways to accomplish the same results. The happiest and most fulfilled women I know are keenly aware of their unique abilities and they understand that each person has access to a different range of talents and abilities.

To complicate matters even further, the commonly accepted view of what constitutes as a talent or unique ability tends to be very narrow. When you think of the word talent, you may first think of *skills*, such as swinging a golf club, changing a diaper, or public speaking. There are so many more ways to be gifted and many lesser known unique abilities.

One of the best tools in my opinion to uncover your talents is the CliftonStrengths assessment from the Gallup organization, the same organization that brings you the opinion polls of the masses.[4] This is an easily accessed online assessment that has been taken by over 33 million people across the world. You may have already taken this assessment through your work or school, but if not, do yourself a favor and check it out. For around $50, this assessment can identify your greatest individual talents, ranking them in order of strength from 1 to 34.

Let this staggering statistic sink in. The odds of someone having the same top 10 talents as you in the same order on this assessment are around 1 in 447 trillion! The odds of meeting someone with all 34 talents in the same order as you are 1 in 295,000,000, 000,000,000,000,000,000,000,000,000! That number is a higher number than the total number of grains of sand on Earth! There is nearly zero chance there could ever be another you who shares your uniquely ordered set of abilities. These statistics prove that you are truly and utterly *unrepeatable!*

For example, my top five strengths according to Gallup definitions are:[5]

- *Achiever: individuals who possess a strong drive to achieve, are naturally productive, and find satisfaction in completing tasks and setting new goals.*
- *Intellection: individuals characterized by their intellectual activity, introspective nature, and appreciation for intellectual discussions.*
- *Connectedness: individuals who have a strong belief in the interconnectedness of all things, seeing meaning and purpose in events and finding value in integrating different parts into a whole.*

- *Input: describes individuals who naturally have a need to collect and archive information, ideas, artifacts, or even relationships, driven by curiosity and a desire to find value in "stuff."*
- *Learner: individuals who have a strong desire to learn and who seek to continuously improve. They usually find the process of learning itself more engaging than the outcome or even the specific subject matter.*[5]

Others may share similar talents but no one I know will share my personal synergistic combination of these gifts. This is both empowering and clarifying, and it naturally peaks my interest to learn more about the talent combination of others.

If you're doubting yourself or having a bad day, remind yourself that important characteristics about you have never before existed nor may ever exist again. If you take only one thing away from this book, *let it be the conviction that the world needs you and your special combination of talents.* Learning your unique abilities and discovering what you do naturally better than others is a major key to finding more purpose and fulfillment after raising kids. Putting your specialized talents to good use often ignites a passion in us that can energize and power us throughout the years to come.

Dr. Brooke and I repeatedly say on our podcast that it's often the small details that make the biggest difference in your life, especially in midlife. Most of you grew extensively in your maturity and experience throughout your teens and twenties which fundamentally shaped you and helped evolve you into the woman you are today. You're not likely to pack that much change into one single decade again. I'll demonstrate my point with the analogy of boiling water. At 211°F, water is just water. But with just one degree of added energy, that temperature rises to 212°F, and suddenly water magically transforms into steam, a whole new physical state with just a little added shift in energy. You don't necessarily need a lot of energy or effort to result in a *big* change in your life. Learning more about your unique abilities is one simple thing that can create a huge ripple effect.

Exercise: Clues to Your Hidden Talents

We've come up with a series of questions as a DIY to help you uncover your unique abilities. I've always resonated with this statement: The quality of your life is determined by the quality of the questions you ask." With the right questions and some honest reflection, you will gain more insight around where you shine.

Do your best to answer the following questions quickly, resisting the urge to give a "fashion show response." At this time, when thinking of your answers, try not to consider the perceptions or thoughts of your family, friends, or community. Just like the goals framework exercise, this isn't the time to stay too grounded in what you currently think is possible for you.

Instead, this is a time to strip back the noise from the outside world and find some inner stillness to tap into your purest self. Listening to your heart and gut is as much a part of this exercise as is thinking with your head, and accessing one or more of these parts of you may take some practice. When you're in the right zone, the answer should come to you without much hesitation. In this state, you can trust that you've uncovered an authentic response. If you're feeling blocked, take a break, change your scenery, or best of all, do something exhilarating or new to you. When you feel more alive and present in the moment, you will naturally be more in alignment with your truest self.

10 Essential Questions for Getting to Know Yourself Again

- If I had unlimited time and/or money, what one or two things would I look back and regret not doing in the next 10–20 years?
- What are the daily or weekly tasks that I look forward to doing the most?
- What have been some of my biggest achievements outside of raising my family?
- What are some things that come naturally to me but seem harder for my friends or family members?

- What tasks feel like absolute drudgery to me when I'm doing them?
- What are some talents that I've been complimented consistently on over the years?
- What are some things I can picture myself doing when I picture my life in the next 10–20 years even if it feels impractical, difficult, or above my skill level?
- What subjects do I yearn to learn more about?
- What are some tasks, activities, or obligations where time seems to fly by, as if I'm in a flow state?
- What would I do for free, if given the opportunity, for pure enjoyment and pleasure?

Dismantle Your Blind Spots

What you don't know about yourself can actually hurt you. As an example, my daughter has a friend at her old school whose mom will tell you, no matter what you're discussing, that she's done the same thing, only better. Do you know the type? Let's call her "Mrs. One-Up Mom." Someone close to her should have pulled her aside by now to point out that her behavior can be off-putting because it appears that she's constantly competing with others.

Do you ever wonder if something you do unknowingly causes others to talk behind your back? That's exactly what was happening with Mrs. One-Up Mom at school functions and football games. When her name was brought up, the other moms would smirk and give knowing looks. I hated that for her!

A tragic truth is that the people closest to us often overlook or ignore such behaviors so they can keep the peace, and the people outside our inner circle may not feel close enough or care enough to intervene. Here's what I think is happening: She's most likely a highly competitive person who actually means well and tries hard to connect to others. I suspect a blind spot for her is measuring her own place against the performance of others. She was a high school athlete, and I believe she's still a very talented competitor who's unaware that she's slipping too many "contests" into everyday conversations. Instead of her yearning to compete passively creeping in where it's unwarranted, she could try a more self-aware approach. For example, she could find ways to bring more games into her every day. She could turn her errands or daily chores at home into a contest (I particularly like the game "Who Can Finish Their Laundry First?"), sign up to train for a beginner triathlon, or hit trivia night every week at the neighborhood bar. It's my belief that by channeling her desire to compete in healthier avenues, she would no longer feel inclined to compete with others verbally.

Once your blind spots are revealed, you, too, can work to find better ways to redirect yourself into healthier channels that bring you more of what you want and stop them from covertly working against you.

Exercise: Identifying Your Personality Blind Spots

The Enneagram personality typing system can help you learn and understand your personality blind spots. We've crafted another helpful quiz for you, this time it's designed to help you find your personal Enneagram type. You can take the quiz at www .lifeafterkids.com/book. Follow the instructions we've included and you'll most likely recognize yourself in your result and accompanying Enneagram type description.

I remember when Dr. Brooke first shared with me her personal a-has upon learning her Enneagram type. As her best friend, I saw a dramatic shift in her at the time. She seemed so much more at peace and relaxed overall. Before that, she'd been struggling with the intrusion of excessive fearful and anxious thinking. Learning that she was an Enneagram 6 had given her some relief she no longer felt alone or there was something deeply wrong. She also felt better equipped to manage her tendency to over-worry through better self-care and better awareness of her needs. She learned that Type 6s have a blind spot in trusting themselves. Typically, they lack those "gut feelings" that many of us rely on.

The Enneagram has been passed down through the ages. No one really knows exactly where it originated from, but it's been used for hundreds of years and in recent years has become popular as a way to better understand behaviors and blind spots. Your Enneagram number gives you clues to your personality blind spots because it points out where you tend to get in your own way.

When I learned I was an Enneagram 1, it explained so much. It explained why I felt the need to be perfect and why I've found myself choosing a façade of perfection even if it comes at a high cost. Before this knowledge, when meeting someone new, I often tried to put forth a perfected version of myself expecting "her" to be more likable than my true self. Of course, that inauthenticity turned many people off, and during that time, I often struggled to make new friends. When I became aware of this blind spot, it spurred a conscious effort to be my true self in new company, flaws and all. The result was I began to build deeper and longer lasting friendships with other women. It was uncomfortable at first and I still catch myself resorting to my old tricks at times. However, owning what I know about my Enneagram type helps me to do better.

There is so much to learn from the Enneagram, from recognizing commonly repeated behavior patterns to spotting the characteristic warning stress signs that can then be avoided. As a woman embarking on a journey for meaning, fulfillment, and enriched relationships, the Enneagram can be a helpful tool to guide you toward better awareness of your blind spots. Below you'll find a brief description of the most common personality blind spots according to each Enneagram type:

Type 1—The Moral Perfectionist Your tendency to high standards can lead you to nitpick and excessively correct others and their approach, when in reality there is more than one way to do something well.

Type 2—The Supportive Helper You can become possessive and jealous when loved ones spend time with other people.

Type 3—The Successful Achiever You see your loved ones as an extension of your image, and you can get upset when others cannot live up to your level.

Type 4—The Romantic Individualist You indulge every emotion you feel, becoming moody and irritable often.

Type 5—The Investigative Thinker You are overly private and can make others feel as if they're invading when in fact they're just trying to show care and concern for you.

Type 6—The Loyal Guardian You tend to test others to see if they're going to stay committed, supportive, and loyal to you.

Type 7—The Entertaining Optimist You can become an escapist when approached with difficult conversations or situations that could cause emotional pain. This can cause others to feel disconnected or dismissed.

Type 8—The Protective Challenger You may attempt to force others to change into what you think they should be rather than respecting who they are.

Type 9—The Peaceful Mediator You numb out when you are overwhelmed by stress, chores, and conflicts and may push off your responsibilities, possibly letting your loved ones down.

Dr. Brooke and I wholeheartedly agree that the Enneagram has been one of the most significant personal discoveries we've learned and applied in midlife. If you're interested in exploring the Enneagram further, we recommend an excellent book on the topic titled *The Road Back to You* by Ian Morgan Cron and Suzanne Stabile.[6] In our opinion, the authors unfold this topic beautifully, making it easy to understand and keeping it tremendously relevant for you.

Putting the Four Ds Together

If you've been following our directions, by now you should be feeling more confident in what you want for your life after kids and more connected to yourself than ever. You should also know the intentional order of these exercises that have been laid out for you is worth noting.

Here's why: When you're feeling down about yourself, you might be tempted to skip to the section on blind spots because you prefer in that moment to wallow in what's not working. We advise you to spend time on your personality blind spots only *after* you've done the work to clarify and gain strength from your new set of values, your compelling life vision, and identifying your unmatched unique abilities.

When you have a crystal clear picture of your Four Ds, confidence comes from having a more solidified idea of who you are and where you're headed in your life. When you are more confident, doors begin to open for you. And more importantly, when you're more confident, you can more easily muster the courage to walk through them.

If you're not seeing it yet, don't despair. The concepts you're learning are meant to build on the ones before. Keep going to see how it all comes together to work for you in the end.

Part II

RESILIENCE

Chapter 4

Simple Strategies for Stress Management

By Dr. Brooke

If you're old enough like me to remember things like plastic Halloween costumes, phones that plugged into walls, and station wagons with third row seats that were rear-facing, then you probably also remember the Slinky. The Slinky, originally made of shiny silver metal, is a helical toy spring popularized for its ability to delight children by being able to go down a flight of stairs end over end on its own. The Slinky is the perfect depiction of what it means to be resilient because it is flexible enough to be stretched, bounced, and pulled, but it's strong enough to go back to its original form. Regardless of the stressor placed on it, the Slinky never loses its shape.

That's exactly what resilience is: the ability to maintain your form regardless of the various ways you are stretched, bounced, and pulled by outside stressors. And in this new phase of life, resilience is precisely what we need to live a vibrant and purposeful life after kids.

The Stress of Midlife

There's no denying this phase of life has its own fair share of stress, and perhaps the kids growing up is even more difficult for us because it's a constant reminder that time is passing by at a rapid rate and we're getting older right along with them. It's not necessarily easy to reach the point in your life when you realize that you likely have the same number of days ahead of you as you do behind you or even fewer days ahead than you do behind. That's already plenty to get the embers of stress flaming in a midlife mom, but just when you think you might be able to stand the heat, more coals are added to the fire. There's health issues to deal with, aging parents to care for, relationships to rebuild, loneliness, and of course, don't forget MENOPAUSE!

Honestly, there's nothing like a good hormone fluctuation to really get you stressed and wanting to pull your hair out. Maybe you're frustrated with me for pointing out all of your woes, and you want to close this book so you can put your stressed out, hot flashing, night sweating self to bed. But please, keep your book open, take a breath, and stay with me because there's more to the story.

This chapter of our life doesn't end on a low and frazzled note merely accepting that the best part of our life is over. We will survive our life after kids, and not only will we survive, we will *thrive* despite all the stress and the ever-changing landscape of midlife. Like the Slinky, we must harness the ability to bounce back from the push and pull of midlife stress that sometimes stretches us more than we would like. So, get ready because this is the most important thing you're going to hear about building resilience in life beyond motherhood:

You will thrive in your life after kids and build more resilience by letting go of the things you cannot control and focusing on the things that you can control.

Maybe that sounds simple and a little too basic, but trust me, there's a lot to unpack here. And it all starts with understanding the things we can't control, followed by focusing on the things we can control.

Strategy for Building Resilience: Control What You Can; Let Go of the Rest

Let's consider for a moment the things we can't control: things like the passage of time, our age, our spouse/partner's actions, our kids' actions, where our kids live, what other people think about us, what other people say to us, and yes even the weather. You'll find that if you choose to dwell on these types of things, you will live a relatively stressed-out life and probably wake up in a bad mood more often than not. And, ironically, all the time we waste worrying and complaining about these things will not actually change them. No amount of worrying about quality time with your kids or the aging process will get your kids to see you more or make you any younger. It's a big waste of your valuable energy to allow the uncontrollable aspects of life to capture your focus and attention. Trying to control every aspect of your life is a surefire way to derail yourself from living your best next chapter.

If I could get back even a quarter of the time that I've wasted worrying about things out of my control, I'd easily get one or two more decades out of my life. As I've already stated, worrying about the uncontrollables is fruitless at best and a joy stealer at worst. Let's instead shift our focus to the things we can control:

- Finding new purpose (see Chapters 2 and 3)
- Partaking in activities and hobbies you enjoy (see Chapter 11)
- Learning new things (see Chapter 11)
- Improving your physical health (see Chapter 6)
- Daily habits and actions
- The words you speak
- Your mindset
- Whom you spend time with (see Chapters 8 and 9)
- Stress management and your emotional health

When you make this list a regular priority in your life, a strange thing happens. You find you have very little time to think about the things you can't control and made you upset in the first place. Suddenly, you find your inner Slinky. If you commit to working on the items listed, you will improve your emotional health and boost your resilience.

Moving forward, the majority of this chapter will address stress management and emotional health for improved resilience, but before we go there, I want to give you one important word of caution:

Do not, I repeat do not, wait until crap hits the fan and you come undone to begin to focus on building emotional health and resilience.

The most important thing I will say to you in this chapter and maybe even this book is be proactive. Take care of yourself, your health, and your emotional balance now so that when hardship does come your way, you'll be more prepared to handle it. It's far easier to continue healthy habits that have been in place when you hit a difficult time than it is to build healthy habits during a difficult time. Do you see the difference? Now let's take a deeper dive into stress management and emotional health.

The Power of Your Words

If we now know that the most important step we can take to thrive in this phase of life is to focus on the things we can control and let go of the things we cannot, then it only makes sense that the first step to stress management and emotional balance would be to adopt habits and tools that help you shift your *mindset*. I happen to have a favorite that I'd like to expand on from the previous list: the words you speak.

Do not discount the power of spoken words and the impact they can have on your emotional health. It will behoove you when building resilience to become very aware of the words you speak. Make a daily practice of shifting your words from negative statements to positive statements. This can help shift your mindset because your brain listens to everything you say. For example, if someone asks you how you're feeling today, instead of saying "I'm absolutely exhausted, I slept terribly last night," shift your words to, "I'm a bit tired due to restless sleep, but I'm sure I'll sleep great tonight."

Likewise, instead of "I haven't heard from my child in ages, they clearly don't care about me much," change it to, "It's been a little bit since I've touched base with my child, but time does go fast, I'm sure they've been busy and will reach out as soon as they have a chance." Instead of over-dramatizing everything with your words, begin to speak more positively about your life and I bet you'll note that you begin to feel more positive too.

Use Affirmations

Affirmations are yet another way that spoken words can build resilience, and they are my second line of attack when working on mindset shifts and stress management. An affirmation is simply a positive thought about your life or yourself that you say out loud repetitively, typically in the morning, but any time of day works. You may say something like "I am healthy. I am strong. I am capable." Notice that the affirmation is written and stated as if it is already happening. In other words, maybe you aren't as healthy as you'd like to be at this point in time; still, you wouldn't have an affirmation that states "I want to be healthy, strong, and capable" Rather say it as if it's happening "I AM healthy, strong, and capable.

There's a couple of other things you should know about affirmations to make them more effective:

- Say them out loud, enthusiastically, and with a smile on your face. Don't hesitate to say them loudly.
- Affirmations are more powerful if you say them while also moving your body. You could hop on a rebounder (mini-trampoline), or do a few squats, jumping jacks, light stretching, or even a little dancing while you say them.

- It will be helpful to write them in a place where you can see them and refer to them often. For example, if you keep a daily planner, write them in the front so you can see them each time you open it. You could also pin a sticky note to your bathroom mirror or write them on your mirror with chalk paint so you see them every morning as you start your day and at night as you end your day. Moreover, if you work at a desk consistently in or outside of your home, it might make sense to keep a list on your desk.

Practicing affirmations is a powerful way to change your mindset and the more you say them, the more effective they will be. Think of it as rewriting the script in your brain. Essentially you are making a practice of replacing negative self-talk with positive words. Sooner or later, with regular practice, you'll not only believe it but will also feel it, too. What's more, as you retrain your brain, it will subconsciously start to push toward adopting other activities and habits that will help you become what you're affirming over yourself. For instance, if you use the previously stated affirmation, "I am healthy, I am strong, I am capable," you will likely find yourself having an easier time choosing healthy foods and moving your body regularly. Similarly, you may find that your attitude in the gym is more positive and motivating.

If you're reading this thinking, "Brooke, this sounds ridiculous, and also a little embarrassing to do," believe me I get it. I've been doing affirmations in my home for years, and my hubby and kids love to tease me by repeating my affirmations in a high-pitched voice. (If there's one thing my kids have gifted me, it's thick skin and the ability to not take myself too seriously.) So, yeah, it probably will feel awkward when you first get started; most new healthy habits do until they become commonplace. But you, like me, will reap the benefits of affirmations if you stay the course.

For example, I've had an extreme fear of flying for over 20 years, so I adopted an affirmation that speaks to that fear. Over the last few years, I began to daily repeat the affirmation, "I am safe. I love to fly. I love to travel," and it's helped me to pretty much kick my fear of flying. That's not to say that I don't get anxious from time to time on a flight or that there aren't other things I do to conquer my fear. But the affirmations have helped, and very often, when I get on a flight, those words come to my mind—"I am safe. I love to fly. I love to travel." In effect, I am retraining my brain. Besides, even though my kids get a good laugh at my expense, they've also seen me doing affirmations for years, they know what it is, and they understand the practice. Hopefully, they've also noticed a positive change in me. Maybe one day, they'll adopt the practice, too, because we all need a mindset shift from time to time.

Something I've adopted more recently along with my affirmations is saying Bible verses that I've memorized out loud directly after my affirmations. This has been of huge benefit to me, and it's strengthening my faith. Consider adding scripture to your affirmations as well if you feel so inclined. Maybe you'd be more comfortable reciting scripture only. That's great, too!

NOTE: To help get you started, we've created a list of helpful affirmations and Bible verses for this phase of life; just go to www.lifeafterkids.com/book to get your list.

Achieve a Calm State by Calming Your Nervous System

Let's turn now from shifting our mind to shifting our nervous system. So many of us are in a constant state of fight-or-flight mode (basically chronic stress) in which our nervous systems are on overdrive. We live our life in anticipation of the ball dropping or that proverbial criminal chasing us down a dark alleyway. For some reason, midlife moms are notorious for having the gift of worst-case scenario thinking. If you deal with anxiety, have digestive distress, struggle with sleep, have headaches, notice an increase in pulse from time to time even at rest, or have palpitations, your nervous system could very well be overactive and stuck in a state of stress. And according to research, stress is the leading cause of sickness in our society.

Knowing that, it's important to manage your stress levels by shifting your nervous system. Plus, your brain is a part of your nervous system, so when you calm your nervous system, you also calm your brain which enables you to think more clearly, manage your life and family changes more easily, and pursue your purpose more fully. There are several tools I use daily to shift my nervous system into a calmer state.

Breath Work

Breath work is a personal favorite of mine because it's simple to do and very effective. I'm prone to getting anxious while driving in the car and nothing calms me as efficiently as breath work. Breath work can even be a great tool to help you calm down before bed.

What works best for me is the 4-7-8 method of breathing. With this method you close your mouth and take four deep breaths in through your nose. Directly after, hold your breath for seven seconds and then exhale for an count of eight through your mouth making a "whoosh sound" as you do. Repeating this for a period of 3–4 minutes minimum will calm your nervous system and help to quiet your brain.

You can do this anywhere, at any time, and I find that the more you practice, the more effective it becomes. Alternate nostril breathing is another great way to calm your nervous system. This method works by directly stimulating the longest nerve in your body, called the vagus nerve. The vagus nerve runs the length of your spine and is responsible for shifting your body from a state of fight or flight to a state of "rest and digest."

NOTE: For a step-by-step guide to alternate nostril breathing and other strategies for stimulating your vagus nerve, go to www.lifeafterkids/book.

Meditation

Meditation is indeed a great way to calm your nervous system and quiet your brain. What you may not know is that meditation doesn't have to be done sitting in a quiet room on the floor, with your legs crossed and your eyes closed as you gently release the word "Om" from your mouth and quiet all your thoughts. If that sounds over-whelming, you are not alone. Take it from a board certified "cannot sit still" woman. Try as I might, I just can't get comfortable with classic meditation. To me, it feels like a chore rather than a beneficial mode of relaxation (no offense to any of our resident yogis and meditators!).

But take heart because if you're like me, you can still reap the benefits of meditation, because anything that brings you into the pre-sent moment and quiets your thoughts can be meditative. Under these guidelines, you might actually be in a meditative state while playing an instrument, crocheting or knitting, working a jigsaw puz-zle, coloring in an adult coloring book, or even walking outside by yourself with no phone: just listening and paying attention to the world around you.

I encourage you to experience the benefits of meditation by partaking in a relaxing activity/hobby or moving your body to calm your nervous system, quiet your mind, and bring you into the present moment, thus lowering stress.

Body Movement

Body movement is another fabulous way to reduce stress and build resilience. Any type of body movement will do. This doesn't have to be in the gym or on the treadmill running several miles. Just aim for moving your body daily. Getting outside first thing in the morning to move adds an even bigger punch because direct sun-light at the start of your day will set your circadian rhythm, aka sleep-wake cycle, thus helping you to fall asleep more easily at night.

All body movement counts when it comes to managing stress and clearing your mind. Walk your dog. Take the stairs. Stretch. Put on some good tunes and dance. Take a hike. Hop on a rebounder. Play pickleball. Find some type of movement you enjoy and do more of it.

And there's nothing that will change a bad mood quicker than taking just five minutes to interrupt negative thoughts by moving your body. Remember this: MOVE YOUR BODY TO CHANGE YOUR MOOD. So, the next time you're feeling sad because you walked past your children's empty room or you're frustrated because they haven't called or texted in a while, don't wallow, move!

Sleep

Sleep is the single most important thing we can focus on to build resilience and reduce our stress. In fact, sleep is when our brain heals, and the deeper, less interrupted sleep you get, the better the healing is.

It bears repeating, a good sleep starts first thing in the morning, so make a habit of going outside when you start your day to get direct sunlight in your eyes. Next, try to get to sleep no later than 10:30/11:00 pm because our best and deepest sleep occurs between 10 pm and 12 am, and most of us need at least 7–8 hours of sleep per night to be our healthiest.

If sleep is a big struggle for you, check out Sean Stevenson's book *Sleep Smarter*, where you'll find 21 ways to improve your sleep for better health. In the meantime, I've listed my top strategies here:

- Turn off electronics at least one hour before bed and consider wearing blue light blocking glasses because the blue light emitted from our devices like phones, tablets, computers, and TVs is known to disrupt the sleep cycle.
- Take magnesium (200–400 mg) before bed for relaxation and deeper sleep. Magnesium is a mineral that almost all of us are lacking due to our food quality. My favorite is magnesium glycinate because it's easily absorbable, doesn't irritate the gut, and is known to help with relaxation and muscle tension.

NOTE: You will know if you are getting too much magnesium as your stool will become loose. If that happens, simply decrease the amount of magnesium you were taking daily. (See the next section.)

- Wear a sleep mask to ensure the room is completely dark (light affects our sleep cycle and the darker your room, the better).

- If your spouse is a snorer, consider ear plugs (they've worked wonders for me and my marriage!).
- Put a drop or two of lavender essential oil on your pillow or the inside of your wrist at bedtime.
- Don't read or watch anything stressful or disturbing in the evening. It could cause anxious feelings and your mind to race making it difficult to unwind and fall asleep.
- Stop eating at least two hours before bed. You will sleep more deeply if your body and brain aren't actively working to digest food when you lie down, and you will help prevent heartburn in the middle of the night.
- Be mindful of alcohol intake. While the research on alcohol can be conflicting, most agree that alcohol is detrimental to hormones and overall health in a myriad of ways. It can even cause sweating and anxiety through the night. Therefore, you should limit alcohol consumption. Personally, I limit my alcohol intake to about once a month on a special occasion. That being said, when it comes to sleep, try not to drink alcohol at least three hours before going to bed. While a drink closer to bed time may seem to help you relax and fall asleep more quickly, it keeps your body from getting into a deep and restful sleep, thus damaging sleep quality.
- Don't discount blood sugar when it comes to waking up through the night and not being able to fall back to sleep. Often, a middle of the night wake up is due to your blood sugar tanking. To keep your blood sugar steady and alleviate the "middle of the night wake ups," be sure to eat a large enough dinner that consists of at least 30 grams of protein.
- For more simple tips for improved sleep quality, go to www .lifeafterkids.com/book.

Finally, many moms fall asleep easily but then wake up with ruminating thoughts that can't be stopped. They wake up thinking about their kids, something they said or wish they had said, or even what they're going to wear the next day. If this sounds like you, consider journaling before bedtime. Stay tuned because this is a topic I'll go into more deeply in the next chapter.

Take Supplements

It's always a good idea to address the cause of your stress and try lifestyle changes before taking something for stress management, even if that something is a supplement. Yet for some of us, our nervous systems are so ramped up that we need a little extra help along the way so we don't go into a tailspin and so we reap the most benefits from the lifestyle habits I mentioned earlier.

Here's the short list of my favorite supplements for stress management and a calmer nervous system:

- *Magnesium,* as mentioned earlier, is known as "the stress mineral", and it is beneficial to the human body in a myriad of ways. It helps to maintain normal nerve and muscle function, supports the immune system, keeps the heartbeat steady, can improve sleep quality, and helps bones remain strong. It also helps with energy and protein production. Magnesium glycinate and magnesium malate are my favorite forms of the mineral, but you could consider magnesium citrate if you have trouble with bowel movements as it's known to help with constipation.
- *L-theanine* is a naturally occurring amino acid found in green tea and black tea. It can also be taken in capsule or tablet form, and may help reduce anxiety and stress while improving sleep. One of the many reasons I love drinking tea is that the combination of caffeine and L-theanine give me a perfect balance of calm energy and focus.
- *Ashwagandha and Rhodiola* are known as adaptogenic herbs because of their ability to help the body adapt to stress. Ashwagandha is an evergreen shrub native to India and the Middle East often used in Ayurvedic medicine. Rhodiola, also known

as golden root or arctic root, thrives in cold weather and high altitudes, growing in Sub-Arctic and Arctic areas. Both herbs share several similarities but ashwagandha is known more for its ability to calm the body down, and Rhodiola is known for its energizing effects.

- *Tulsi* (also known as holy basil) is an aromatic perennial plant that is native to tropical and subtropical regions of Asia, Australia, and the western Pacific. Tulsi is known for health benefits, such as stress reduction and improved digestion. It can be taken in capsule or liquid form, but I prefer the tea, and I drink it every time I am traveling by plane to keep me calm and reduce anxiety. For me, tulsi has been the most impactful supplement for managing stress and calming my nervous system. I notice a calming effect shortly after drinking the tea.
- *Passion flower* is a climbing vine with white and purple flowers. The chemicals in passion flower have calming effects. Passion flower can be used in capsule, tincture, or tea form and is known for its effects on the nervous system, reducing anxiety and improving sleep.
- *B. Subtilis* is a type of probiotic that some research has shown to positively influence mood and potentially reduce anxiety and depression. This type of probiotic has been very effective for me. I prefer to take it in spore form because it is shelf stable, has no expiration date, and cannot be broken down by your stomach acid before it ever reaches the intestinal tract.

You can learn more and shop our favorite brands here: www .lifeafterkids/book.

Please note, it's prudent to make changes to your eating habits as well if you're really struggling with stress and emotional balance. Remember that if your diet consists of mostly garbage, you are likely to feel mostly like garbage. The best and easiest place to start is by limiting sugar intake and replacing processed foods with whole healthy foods (more on this in Chapter 7). Moreover, one of the simplest things you can do for overall health and also stress management is to keep yourself fully hydrated by drinking up to 50% of your body weight in ounces of water per day. I have found that if I am feeling anxious or fatigued, drinking a large glass of water is often the remedy. Be sure to drink your daily intake of water before 7 pm, as drinking too much after this time could interrupt your sleep with the need to go to the bathroom.

You Are Not Alone

I've spent most of my adult life learning about and working on ways to manage stress and build resilience, not only for my patients and clients but also for myself. I know that every tool and strategy I've mentioned in this chapter works because I use them regularly, and if you make them a daily habit, they can work for you too.

Anxiety and emotional imbalance have been a struggle of mine for years, rearing their ugly heads for the first time in college and subsequently ebbing and flowing through adulthood. I remember distinctly flying home from my 40th birthday celebration in the Bahamas and talking to Dr. Lynne on the plane about how excited I was for the next phase of life. I related that I was looking forward to my kids getting older and my husband and I having more time to travel and have adventures. I noted that I was anticipating the years ahead excitedly with older kids and I was looking forward to focusing on my career.

As life would have it, just a few short weeks after making those statements, the bottom dropped out of the loaded bag that was my life. I lost a family member and a very close family friend within weeks of each other, my husband and I became primary caretakers of his 93-year-old blind grandmother, and I started a new business.

At that time, I wasn't doing any of the strategies that I just broke down for you except for being mindful of the foods I ate. And for a while, I coasted through those months of chaos and stress.

I was in survival mode. And people needed me. In some ways it was an adrenaline rush and I felt a bit like superwoman. But here's the ironic thing. When the dust settled, when my life slowly began to normalize, and when my body knew it was safe to take a breath while letting its guard down, I fell apart. And when I say fell apart, I mean broken emotional glass all over the floor.

I couldn't sleep. I'd wake up in the middle of the night in a full-on panic attack, drenched in sweat with my heart pounding out of my chest. I had heart palpitations. I had trouble driving. I once had a panic attack so bad that I fell to the ground and almost passed out right in the middle of the checkout line at Whole Foods. At my worst, I had myself so convinced I had a heart problem that I was afraid to go up the stairs in my house. This led to a comprehensive health and cardiology exam.

I remember very clearly sitting in my cardiologist's office as he went over all the testing and procedures I had completed. Everything was normal, he said. My heart looked great. There was nothing wrong with it except stress, anxiety, and maybe a little hormonal imbalance. I felt as if I had a new lease on life. I had been so convinced for so long that there was something physically wrong with me that I really felt like I had a second chance at life. And I didn't want to blow it.

So, I did what any woman in my position would do. I called my mother! Yep. I sure did. I sat there in the parking lot of my office directly after my doctor's appointment, on the phone with my mother to discuss my new lease on life. Unbelievably, I found out during that conversation that my mom had dealt with very similar issues when she was about my age. It was so freeing, encouraging, and empowering to know that I was not alone and that I could move on from all of this darkness just as my mom had.

Turns out, this is a big part of why I currently do what I do. It's because moms need to have these real and honest conversations. We need to listen to each other, support each other, help each other to build resilience, and become the best versions of ourselves. We need to know that we are not alone in our struggles.

I cannot tell you how many times we've heard from moms in our community, "Thank you so much for saying that. I thought I was the only one." When we know we're not alone in our struggle, whether that's anxiety, emotional imbalance, feeling lost or stuck, menopause, or just plain missing the crap out of our kids, it not only comforts us but also helps us to be more gracious to ourselves and more motivated to move forward, knowing we're going to be ok.

As I reflect on my personal story, I draw parallels to our current phase of life. I related to you that I powered through that busy and stressful time without much, if any, focus on stress management, and it didn't catch up with me until the chaos subsided at which point I began to fall apart. I wonder now if this isn't far off from what happens to a mom as her kids leave home.

See, we spend so many years running the marathon of mommy life. We cook. We clean. We run a laundromat. We tutor. We organize and schedule the calendar. We chauffeur, carting our kids everywhere they need to go. We shop. We're party planners. We're volunteers and coaches. And we're travel guides. All of these roles leave very little time for our own self-care and stress management. We simply speed through our child-raising years in "adrenaline-junky" survival mode until the kids grow up and become independent. They leave home and our lives start to quiet down as the dust of mothering 24-7 settles.

Then, and only then, do our bodies and minds realize they can let their guard down and breathe again. And in that place of solitude and quiet, we fall apart a little bit or even a lot.

Fortunately, you are capable of building resilience and mending yourself and your fractured heart just as I did. The tools discussed in this chapter will help you manage stress. They will enable you to be more calm, grounded, and clear-headed, which will lead to better energy and more motivation for you to pursue your purpose and live a more fulfilling life after kids. And if you're worried about what your relationship with your kids will look like down the road or you're concerned about the time you'll spend with them or the amount of regular communication you'll receive from them, focus on channeling your inner Slinky.

Give your kids the gift of a mom who's living a well-balanced, centered, grounded, happy, and meaningful life. Watch and see how it draws them to you. Watch and see how it draws others to you. Because at the end of the day, everybody loves a Slinky!

Chapter 5

Embracing What Is

By Dr. Brooke

It's a beautiful, sunny, albeit crisp Thursday morning in June, the kind that reminds me of why I love living in New England. I take slow, quiet steps into my nine-year-old son's room to gently nudge him out of sleep so he can get ready for school and make the bus on time. As his long, thick eye lashes begin to flutter over his eyes indicating to me that he is shaking off sleep, I say what all moms have said hundreds of times over the years, "Good morning, love; time to get up for school. Get dressed and come downstairs for breakfast."

He sits up slowly and begins to stretch, and as I leave his room, I proceed toward one of my biggest mom regrets in life. Because, just before I head to the stairs, I turn and flippantly tell him, "Oh, by the way, you didn't make the travel baseball team, the coaches emailed us last night." And if that wasn't bad enough, I finish with, "Get moving so you don't miss the bus." At that moment, as moms often do, I went from energetically prepping for a beautiful spring morning to my heart breaking open inside of me because suddenly, my beautiful sweet boy was looking at me with a swell of tears pouring down his face.

Major mom fail—I never would have guessed my son, who was and has always been an independent, strong, and self-confident kid, would be so wrecked by the news of not making that team, especially because it wasn't his primary or even favorite sport. In fact, he had decided to try out for the team because he loved to be active and loved competition but mostly because all of his friends were avid ball players and he wanted to spend his summer playing with them.

Honestly, the kid really didn't even care much about baseball, which is why I so casually broke the news to him that morning. However, what I neglected to consider as a mom was how wrapped up my son was in his identity as an athlete, even at that age, and how focused he was on spending the summer playing and competing with his friends. For him, the heartache wasn't over the thing itself—making the actual team—it was that his view of himself and his expectations for his life at that time did not align with his reality. The disconnect between what he thought he wanted and absolutely needed for his life and what was actually happening released a torrential downpour of emotions, causing his tears to flow and my heart to break.

Isn't it crazy how our emotions and feelings are so wrapped up in our children and what's happening in their world and in their heart? It's as if our hearts beat succinctly with their heart beat. And it's not just when the kids are little. In fact, in my own life, I would say that the older my kids have gotten, the more strongly I feel their emotions—the good and the bad.

While writing this book, another of my three sons was preparing to leave home for college for the first time. He and I had sat together for a solid two hours filling out online surveys for roommates and studying available dorms so he could submit his top eight room requests in order of importance to the head of housing on his college campus. A few months later, he found out he got placed in a dorm that wasn't even on his list, and in his opinion, one of the worst dorms on campus. Oh, the drama that ensued. Oh, how my mama's heart pitter-pattered with his.

In a similar state to his brother from my earlier story, what was happening in real life was not at all aligned with his expectations. And he was so upset that his ideal was not met that he missed the benefits of his situation—things like he would be closer to his classes and, because he had a shared bathroom, the school would be responsible for keeping it clean, so he wouldn't have to.

Managing Expectations and Ending Comparisons

Let's face it, as moms, we have so many expectations and emotions to manage. Coping with and advising our kids is one thing, but keep in mind we're also managing our own lives and shortcomings. If we're being honest, we've all been in the same place as our kids more times than we'd like to remember.

When we were younger, it may have been devastation over not having the same metal Strawberry Shortcake lunch box and thermos as the girl sitting next to us at lunch. Fast-forward a few years and it was sitting at home alone on a Friday night while two of your friends were having a sleepover together. Later still, it was not getting the job, the house, or the "fill in the blank" that you wanted.

And now that the kids are older, we have even more expectations for our lives, don't we? For example:

- We want our kids to live nearby.
- We want to be actively involved in their lives.
- We want to have a strong relationship with their spouse or significant other.
- We want our own strong friendships and connections.
- We want a solid romantic relationship.
- We want the ability to travel and the freedom to pursue activities we love.

And as if the expectations we place on our own lives weren't enough, we also look around at the lives of other moms in our community and play the comparison game. Suddenly, talking to our adult kids every week or so isn't nearly enough because Sue down the street talks to her kid every single day. The amount of expectations we place on our lives and the ideals that we strive for are endless. You would think we'd be at an age where we would be past all this, but in some ways, in this phase of life, the expectation and comparison might actually be worse, probably because we recognize the finiteness of time and feel a tremendous push to finally get our life right.

There is, however, something to be said for realizing that life is short and, therefore, learning to enjoy the present moment while being joy-filled right where we are in life. Please don't misconstrue what I am suggesting here. Understand that in this phase of life, you should have a focus on writing an amazing next chapter. It's the primary reason Dr. Lynne and I are writing this book. We urge you and the rest of the moms in our community to actively pursue more purpose for a more fulfilling life now that your kids are grown. And, creating change through setting goals and having expectations for your life is a very important part of growing yourself and living more purposefully.

On the other hand, if you get too caught up in the expectations you have for your life or you're constantly and consistently chasing an ideal that may not even be attainable, you will do yourself two big disservices. First, you'll miss the joys of the present moment and second, you'll rob yourself of happiness, because:

> *The single best way for you to create unhappiness in your life after kids is to have a disconnect between the expectations for your life and the way your life actually is.*

So, is the answer to simply set lower expectations for your life so you're never disappointed and don't experience the unhappiness of disconnect between what you intended and what really is? Absolutely not. Lowering your expectations is a direct path to living a subpar life. You should dream big for your life. You should use the Life after Kids Goals Framework. And you should adopt a growth mindset.

Likely, if you don't feel at least slightly unsettled or a hint of discontent, you won't be prompted to ask more from yourself and your life and you won't become all that you could be. But you need to have a few practical tools in place to ensure that, as you work toward recreating your life now that your kids are grown, you don't get sidetracked by constantly longing for things to be different or wishing you had more. To build resilience and really thrive in this phase of life you must have a balance, albeit it delicate, between not settling—asking more of yourself and your life and finding joy and contentment right where you are. In the following sections, I'll discuss four useful ways to keep that balance, while putting an end to comparison.

Journaling

If you spend a lot of time in your head, worrying about things you can't control and wishing that various aspects of your life were different, allow me to introduce you to journaling. It just may be your best friend moving forward.

Journaling is a practice that allows you to rid your mind of everything it's ruminating on by writing it in a journal, a notebook, or a piece of paper. The act of writing down negative thoughts and worries allows you to process the thought and remove it from your mind. Keep a journal on your bedside table and write down everything that is bothering you—that's right, anything and everything. Put your pen to paper and just start writing. Write the things you're concerned about, afraid of, angry over—anything that gets you stressed. Be sure to include discontentment and things in your life that you wish were different. Don't worry about punctuation or grammar; just write whatever comes to mind.

Doing this activity at night is particularly helpful if you have difficulty falling asleep or if you wake up in the middle of the night because you can't quiet your mind or stop thinking. When you're done writing, you can take it up a notch by tearing the piece of paper out of your notebook, ripping it into pieces and throwing it away. This symbolic act will let your brain know that you've processed the thoughts, you're done with them, and it's time to move on. It can be very cathartic. Often, the things that are bothering us or causing us angst are embedded in our subconscious and we aren't even aware of them. We have no idea that these things are at the root of how we're feeling. Journaling can help bring these problematic thoughts to the forefront of our brain, allowing us to address them and process them.

From there, we can choose what we'll do with what we've written: accept it or do something about it. Keep in mind that almost always, acknowledging the problem is half the battle in the war of living a vibrant life after kids. Journaling will help you acknowledge and process underlying problems of discontentment.

Gratitude Practice

Another powerful journaling practice is to take a moment at the start or end of the day and write 3–5 things you are grateful for. This practice does three things:

- First, it will create a shift from a negative to positive state of mind because you are teaching your brain to focus on the things that are going well in your life, and the things that make you happy. Research shows that you cannot be in a state of gratitude and fear or anger at the same time. So, when you take a few minutes to think about and write things you are grateful for, you shift away from negativity and move toward happiness.
- Second, it will stop you from comparing yourself and your life to the moms around you because gratitude practice shifts your focus away from the things your wish were different and towards the things you already have in your life to be grateful for—things that are going well.
- Third, the more you practice listing gratitudes regularly, the more your brain will daily look for things to be grateful for. You'll find yourself noticing little joys as you move through your day.

Your gratitude list could include something big like "I finally reached my goal in the gym today" or "I had an amazing long weekend away with my besties." But it could also be something small like "The sky was a beautiful blue today," "I loved the way the wind sounded as it whistled through the trees during my walk," or "I had a great chat with my son/daughter today." Big or small, it all counts, and it all has the power to transform your mind and reduce your stress.

I've seen the power of gratitude practice play out often in my own life. For example, through most of my adulthood, I've often found it difficult to connect with and build friendships with other women. I guess it's because I was raised with brothers and I was always so close to my dad. Whatever the case, relationships with other women just don't come naturally to me. In more recent years, I've found myself yearning for deeper connections with other women, especially now that my kids are older and not occupying most of my time.

To make matters worse, I've compared my own life with other moms I know who have an enormous amount of girlfriends, and I've longed not just for more friends but for a tight knit community of other moms that I can do life with and laugh with, sharing the ups and downs of growing older together. But thus far, friendships and groups such as these have eluded me. And would you agree that the older you get, the harder it becomes to make new friends, and harder still to insert yourself into already established friend groups?

If you'll press pause on this conversation for a moment, you'll note two things that we've been talking about are taking place here. Number one, the expectation I have for my life (more friendships/community) and the reality of my life are not the same. There's an obvious disconnect between the way I expect my life to be and the way it actually is. Not only that, comparing myself and my life to other moms and their friend groups magnifies the disconnect of what I want in my own life. And as already mentioned, when what you expect from your life is out of alignment with how your life actually is and when you compare your life to other peoples, you are setting yourself up for unhappiness. I wish I could tell you that's not been the case in my own life, but I would be lying if I said this disconnect has not caused me to be unhappy and upset from time to time. But journaling/processing and gratitude practice have helped me tremendously.

Remember when I told you that acknowledging and understanding the problem is half the battle? Well the same rang true for me in this case. It required me taking the time to think, process, and even write about what was going on in my life before I realized that "the friendship dilemma" was the cause of discontent. Honestly, the act of typing this now to share with you feels extremely empowering and cathartic, so don't discount the importance of processing, writing, and journaling in your own life.

What's more, if you don't feel like you have anyone to discuss your struggle with, journaling is a great substitute. It gives you the opportunity to share how you're feeling and unload it from your mind. It's an outlet for venting when you feel there is nobody else to vent to. It's like having a conversation with yourself. And by the way, you should be your own best friend, so whom better to talk to than you!

Then there are gratitudes. They've been one of the most useful and helpful tools in my life for managing emotional well-being. And in this particular situation, they were like a warm, comforting hug. See, I could have spent all my time focusing on how sorry I felt for myself because I didn't have more friendships and connection, but all that would do is make me more miserable. So, instead, I shifted to reminding myself to be grateful for everything related to friendship that I already have in my life.

For example, I've had the privilege of sharing life with Dr. Lynne for over 20 years, and she probably knows me better than anyone else. And even though we don't live close to each other, we are blessed to have the ability to see each other and travel together regularly. I have my cousin Kirsten who adores me and my family and loves to visit from Detroit. My husband is like a best friend and he gives great advice. Plus, my brother recently married the woman of his dreams who also happens to be the sister of my dreams. I've waited my whole life to have a sister!

I share all of this with you because I want you to have perspective for yourself and an understanding of how journaling and gratitudes can be of benefit. Start the same activities in your own life. Right now, right where you are, stop what you're doing. Pull out a blank piece of paper and grab a pen. Before you start writing, sit quietly for a few moments and allow yourself to think freely and feel your feelings. Are there any emotions that bubble up? Write about them. Keep writing, don't lift your pen, just get it all out. Eventually, you'll uncover a cause of misalignment or discontent in your life that you may not have even been aware of. Now take some time to think on related things you already have that you can be grateful for and write those things down. Remember to take time daily to review this list and make a regular habit of listing things you are grateful for each day so you can reap all the benefits I've mentioned, and you can begin to feel more joyful in your life.

Goals Check-In

Once you've practiced journaling and gratitudes and become more aware of aspects of your life that aren't the way you hoped they would be, you can take steps to change them by setting goals for your life. Here's where the Life after Kids Goals Framework comes in.

But remember, as helpful as the framework is for dreaming big and reaching for more in your life now that the kids are grown, this chapter is all about finding contentment and joy right where you are. Fortunately, the Life after Kids Goals Framework can be useful in this vein as well, especially if you are prone to never feeling satisfied or comparing your life to others. While this unhealthy cycle can be stopped or lessened with journaling and gratitude practice, it's always a good idea to have other tools in your tool box.

NOTE: Another favorite tool is a monthly and quarterly check in with the Life after Kids Goals Framework (which you can download at https://www.lifeafterkids.com/book). This check-in is such a simple thing, but it has a huge impact. It's worth it to point out, yet again, that it's almost always the little things that end up being the big things.

A regular check in with your goals framework is essentially just as it sounds. Once a month and quarterly, you will take time to sit with your framework and reassess your goals. As you sift through each goal category, notice any goal that has been achieved and cross it off. Be sure to celebrate your win. If you find others that you have not achieved but no longer serve you, go ahead and cross those off as well.

Please note, that it's completely fine to decommit to a goal, and it doesn't make you weak or a quitter. Life can change quickly and sometimes in ways you could not have been prepared for. Considering this, it's common to come across goals that no longer serve you while completing a check-in. Let's face it, if you are committed to a vibrant next phase of life, then you are changing as a person, and who you are a month from now or three months from now may not be the same person you are today. It stands to reason then that, as you move through life, some goals you had set for yourself will no longer serve you. And when you notice this, during a goals check in, give yourself a hug or a warm pat on the back because it means you are becoming more self-aware.

One word of caution here, just be sure that before you cross that goal off completely you take a moment or two to be sure you're removing it because it's not serving you and not because it scares you or it doesn't seem attainable. Remember, growth happens when we push ourselves outside of our comfort zone. (More on this in Chapter 10.)

As you can imagine, a goals check-in will 100% aid you in achieving your goals, but it will also help with your emotional balance and resilience. Because when you start the process by crossing off the goals you've completed, you show yourself how far you've actually come, and if you were feeling stuck or unsatisfied, crossing off those goals will help get you unstuck and will turn your frown upside down.

Sometimes, we focus so much on the future or the big picture that we lose track of all that we've already accomplished. Checking in with your goals will solve that problem for you because it will help you embrace and celebrate what already is! Not to mention, when you intentionally dedicate your time, energy, and focus to your own goals by checking in with them and acting on them, suddenly you have very little time to play the comparison game with other moms. It's a double win!

Ask Whom You Want to Be, Not What You Want to Have

The next exercise that I'm going to walk you through can be a real game changer if you find yourself unhappy due to a disconnect between what you want from your life and what you actually have. But before we dive in, there's something I want you to consider. When you find yourself in a rut, would you agree that it's typically due to things you don't HAVE? For example, you don't HAVE enough money saved for retirement. You don't HAVE enough time with your grown kids? You don't HAVE the perfect relationship. You don't HAVE the ability to travel as much as you'd like. You don't HAVE enough friends.

When using tools like the goals framework, you are focusing on what you want to have in your life. Once again, that is a good thing, and it will enable you to recreate your next phase of life while finding more purpose. But if that is your primary or only focus, you will probably, at one time or another, feel let down, disconnected, and thus, unhappy. That's why you need the tool of "determining whom you want to be" in your tool box.

With this exercise, you will pull out a piece of paper or a journal and begin to think about and then write who you want to be. This exercise is not addressing all the things you want to have in your life—that's an external job. Rather, this is an internal job. Instead, we're going to focus on your emotions and on creating the feelings you want in your life.

Do you want to be a positive person who lights up a room when they walk into it, always with a smile on your face. Write it. Perhaps you want to be a kind and caring woman who always has an encouraging word or a friendly hug. Write that. Or do you see yourself as vibrant and energetic, able to sweep others up in your energy, motivating them to take action. Again, put it on paper. Ask yourself what kind of a mother, friend, spouse, daughter, aunt, sister, community member, WOMAN you want to be and write it. You get to decide whom you want to be in your life after kids, and it's never too late for change! (For more on this, check out Greg Harden's book, *Stay Sane in an Insane World*.)

Be sure to keep this paper handy and refer to it often, especially when you're feeling a little down or longing for things to be different in your life. Remember, that real joy, joy that lasts, doesn't come from the fleeting things we're all chasing after. Yes, the career, the activity, the friends, the shiny jewelry, the new shoes, whatever it is, they feel good in the moment, but they aren't what brings lasting happiness into our life. And sure, having your kids close by and getting to spend regular time with them, or traveling the world, or having regular girls nights out, and amazing date nights with your spouse will always put a smile on your face and in your heart. But these things are often out of your immediate control.

Try as you might, you will never be able to control what other people do, and if you're expecting them to be the full source of your joy, you're going to come up short. For emotional balance and true happiness in your life after kids, you must focus on the things you can control. You do have agency over yourself. You can control your own actions and you can control who you choose to be in this world even if you can't control what you have or what other people do.

The Power of Finding Joy in the Life You're Already Living

With age, loving yourself becomes more and more important, but for some reason, it seems that midlife women still find so many reasons not to love themselves or their lives. I want to take a moment to encourage you that you are already enough, and right now even in this moment, you have so many things to be grateful for. Sometimes, you just need to take a step back from the business of life, the never-ending comparison to others, and the unattainable ideals you set to see it. What a gift we give to ourselves and our kids when we find joy in the life we're already living and love for whom we already are, while still reaching for new goals and further growth.

The ironic thing about taking the time to be present and grateful for what you already have while appreciating who you've already become and getting clear on who you want to be, is that it kicks the door wide open to better relationships and more attainable goals for your life. Because when you can be grateful and content right where you are, you will be more emotionally balanced, which will lead to clearer thinking and more energy to focus on what you want to have. You may also find more free time to focus on new things to do with your life because you won't be spending precious time longing for things to be different and comparing your life to the life of others.

Now that we're in a phase of life in which the age of our kids is showing us daily how fast time goes and how we can never get it back once it's gone, learning to not waste our time on unproductive and often detrimental things is one of the greatest blessings any midlife mom can give to herself.

Chapter 6

Physical Health Is Emotional Health

By Dr. Brooke

Would you agree that as a young adult, you didn't spend much time, if any, contemplating your health or considering any necessary risk assessment? Think about it. Teenagers are notorious for feeling unstoppable, adopting a mindset of "that would never happen to me," rarely considering the consequences of their actions. Moreover, as a teenager, you're so excited about growing up and being independent that you wish the clock would move faster.

Similarly, twentysomethings are just plain living their best idiotic life, many abusing their bodies with too much late night fun, not having much of a care in the world. Evidenced in my own life with riding on the back of motorcycles without a helmet, drinking coffee in the evening by the potful to pull all-nighters during grad school, and living for a solid year on nothing but pickles, pretzels, and ramen noodles.

Sometimes, I wish I could go back and tell my younger self that everything I'm doing to my body will affect how I live later in life. (If only I had a friend in Marty McFly and Doc Brown.) But, since we can't go back in time, let's keep moving forward. Next on the horizon is your 30s, leading you to take advantage of your body and health in different ways. You're now growing your family and maybe also focused on work and a career. This means sleep deprivation, a good deal of stress, and running yourself ragged, often relying on heaps of caffeine just to get through the day. Still, most of us probably gave little thought to what we were actually doing to our body and how it would affect us in the long term. But when we enter our 40s a shift takes place.

When you hit 40, at least for me, you become more and more aware of just how fleeting life is. Hormone flare ups, anxiety (likely from a lot of the stupid things done in youth), and changes in body composition are a blinking road sign warning us to slow down due to curves in the road up ahead. As we ponder the finiteness of life coupled with not being as preoccupied with kids that require our full attention, our focus turns not only towards finding new purpose, but also to our age, our health, and what we can do to stay well. Some of us may adopt a somewhat hedonistic "eat and drink for tomorrow we die" outlook, while the rest of us will decide we want to do whatever we can to make sure we don't just have quantity of years in life, but also quality years as well.

The question I pose is "What good is it to live until the age of 80 or even 90 if your body is breaking down, you cannot live independently, and are unable to enjoy your life?" How many elderly people do you know who are living a large portion of their life in pain and frustration? Unfortunately, I know far more than I care to admit. In this phase of life, it's a constant reminder to be grateful for your health and to take the steps necessary now to live a vibrant life later.

You Have Control Over Your Health

I hope you are well aware that you have agency over your health. Your body is yours and you are in control of it as well as your health, meaning, how you age isn't just left up to chance, good genes, or good luck. This is an important concept for all of us to understand and it should make us feel powerful in our body, motivating us to take the tactical steps needed to ensure that to the best of our ability we are doing what we can to improve our health and longevity.

Yes, obviously there are aspects to life that are out of our control, as with our health, but in most cases, the lifestyle habits we adopt day in and day out have a major impact on our overall health, and that can be in a positive or negative way. (If you don't believe me, take a look at the field of epigenetics, which is the theory and study of how your behaviors and environment can cause changes that affect the expression of your genes. For more on epigenetics, check out the book by David A Sinclair, PhD, *Lifespan: Why We Age—and Why We Don't Have To*.)

Bear in mind that doing nothing for your health and wellness is a choice in and of itself. At a minimum, we should aim for not having a negative impact on our health, but in the best-case scenario, it's important to do what we can to have a positive effect that will increase our longevity. The list of things you can do to improve your health and support your longevity is longer than you might imagine. The good news is that most of these tactics are simple and easy to implement. The hardest part is just getting started, but I'm hoping that after you finish this chapter, you'll get started right away.

The most important things you can do for your physical health and longevity are as follows:

- Prioritize sleep.
- Manage stress.
- Adopt a positive mindset.
- Move your body.
- Eat clean and healthy foods.
- Detox periodically by sweating out the toxins.
- Balance your hormones.

The first three items on this list have already been discussed. In Chapter 4, we discussed sleep and stress management, and in

Chapter 5, mindset. If you need more details and practical tips regarding better sleep, stress management, or procuring a positive mindset, refer to those chapters. We'll discuss the rest of the list in the following sections.

At this point, I would be remiss if I didn't begin our discussion on physical health and longevity by pointing you back to your mental health and emotional balance, because mental health is physical health. You literally cannot separate the two. Your brain is the most important organ in your body and it controls every single thing that takes place in it via the nervous system. Your brain even controls your immune system (which is responsible for keeping you healthy) via the nervous system. The brain, the nervous system, and the rest of your body are so closely intertwined that if either are functioning subpar or under too much stress, your physical health may begin to suffer. It's the reason why researchers and statistics show that stress is the number one cause of disease.

Please recognize that not only is your emotional and mental health of utmost importance for productively pursuing your purpose beyond motherhood, but it also has a direct correlation to your overall physical health and longevity. Similarly, if you are physically unwell or suffering from a debilitating physical sickness, it's not uncommon to also become anxious or even depressed. And if you're lacking in energy or dealing with brain fog (both signs of insufficient physical health), you'll never be able to fully pursue new purpose and passion which could lead to a less than ideal second phase of life. In short, mental and emotional health are physical health, and both are required to live your best, fullest, and most meaningful life after kids.

You'll recall from Chapter 4 that I discussed moving your body daily for improved mental health and emotional balance. The type of body movement we need to talk about now is more focused on building physical strength that will improve longevity and independence, flexibility to keep you mobile, and specific exercises for your posture and spinal health.

Body Movement: Physical Strength, Flexibility, and Posture

Building physical strength in midlife is non-negotiable for every woman that aims to thrive in this phase of life and age vibrantly. Lifting weights or bodyweight training should be done several times a week in order to build muscle and strength. Building muscle is beneficial to you for several reasons. More muscle mass not only helps your metabolism, but it will also help keep your skin tight, and provide protection to your bones and joints from injury.

Plus, building your muscle will keep you strong and independent. I don't know about you, but as I age, I want to be able to continue to do things for myself, things like lifting my own grocery bags and being responsible for my own luggage when I travel. Exercises like weight lifting and bodyweight training will ensure that you strengthen your muscles, while keeping you leaner and healthier in life.

As Dr. Lynne says, there's nothing like pushing yourself in the gym in ways that you didn't know were possible to really make you feel powerful and in control of your own life. It is remarkable how pushing yourself in your workouts can translate to more confidence in yourself and your capabilities in the rest of your life and that includes any goals or new purpose that you are working on.

If you haven't already adopted a weight training routine, I encourage you to get started today. Joining a gym would be a great place to start. Most will provide you with a trainer that will help you get the lay of the land in the weight room, instructing you on all of the equipment so you don't feel overwhelmed. If that doesn't appeal to you, consider taking group weight lifting or barre classes. Most gyms offer these types of classes. Keep in mind that this could also be a fantastic place to make new connections and meet new friends.

Personally, I prefer to do my workouts in the comfort of my own home and if you feel the same way, you're in luck, because there are a variety of classes you can stream online and there are plenty of virtual trainers/coaches you can work with. The good news about strength training is that it doesn't typically require a lot of space or expensive equipment to be effective.

Similarly, flexibility and posture exercises can be done from the comfort of your own home with very little money needed for equipment. These types of exercises are commonly overlooked usually because our time is limited and we'd rather spend it doing things that seem more important to our health and our body image like cardio and weight training. But believe me when I say, flexibility and postural exercises are every bit as important as any other exercise you make time for.

For example, you must maintain your flexibility in order to continue to do day to day tasks throughout life as you age. All of us want to be able to bend down and tie our own shoes or sit on the floor and play with our grandkids, and activities such as these require flexibility. Simple hamstring stretches in which you sit on the floor with your legs straight in front of you and then you fold over to get your hands as close to your toes as possible will go miles to keep you flexible and mobile. Plus, loose hamstrings are a very important part of maintaining a healthy, pain-free lower back. You can also loosen your hamstrings along with many other muscles to maintain flexibility by using a foam roller and an infinity (double massage ball) exercise roller. For more information on flexibility exercises and equipment got to www.lifeafterkids.com/book or go to www.lifeafterkids.com/podcast and listen to Episode 68 of our podcast, released on 28 August 2024.

Foam rollers are also very useful for helping you maintain healthy posture as you age. By simply laying on a large foam roller face up with the top of your head resting at one end of the foam roller and your pelvis resting on the other end, arms stretched on the ground at either side, you can open up tight chest muscles, bring your spine into better alignment, avoid rounding in your shoulders, and even calm your nervous system.

Working on your posture as you age is important for many reasons. First, the better your posture, the healthier your spine will be with less risk of arthritis and pain. Second, when you stand up taller and straighter you not only look better, but you feel better too. And finally, when your head is over your shoulders where it should be, instead of too far forward, you'll have less neck pain, better energy, and less risk of headaches. Postural exercises are simple and easy to do, requiring very little energy. The key is to practice them regularly and often so that they are effective. They work because you are slowly retraining your muscles with repetition, and that takes time and effort. For more information on postural exercises, go to www.lifeafterkids.com/book.

Eating Clean for Midlife Health and Longevity

We cannot have a full discussion on physical health and longevity in this phase of life if we don't include the food we eat along with exercise. And what you may not know is that what you eat is every bit as important to your health and weight as any exercise you will ever do. You simply cannot neglect one for the other.

That being said, while it is so important to move your body daily and weight train regularly, you'll improve your health and change your body more effectively by maintaining healthy eating habits along with regular exercise.

Earlier, in Chapter 4, I mentioned that if you eat mostly garbage, you're going to feel like mostly garbage, and it's worth repeating again. What I really want you to understand and own is that the food you eat goes far beyond your weight or how you look, as it directly affects your physical health and, of course, your emotional health too. Because we just discussed the importance of building muscle later in life with weight training, we should also talk about how you can support your muscle mass with the foods you eat. And the single most important food you can eat for longevity, healthy hormones, metabolism, and yes, muscle mass, is protein.

I cannot stress enough just how important protein is to a midlife woman's overall health, and sadly, most of us are not getting enough protein in our daily diet. For starters, the by-products of protein (amino acids) are a necessary building block for many important things in your body like hormones, neurotransmitters (brain chemicals), enzymes, and cellular function. In other words, lack of protein and thus amino acids can eventually lead to problems with hormone imbalance, brain function, and cellular health. And if that's not enough of a reason to get you to eat more protein, consider that protein also fires your metabolism, keeps you fuller longer, and builds your muscle (you already know the importance of muscle in your body).

I believe, as do many other health care providers, that women over 40 require even more protein in their diet than they did at a younger age in order to stay healthy. To maximize muscle growth and prevent muscle loss, you should be eating 0.7 grams of protein per ideal body weight daily (for more information on this, check out Dr. Gabrielle Lyon's Book *Forever Strong*). Ideally, I strive for about 1 gram of protein per ideal body weight a day. That means, if your ideal body weight is about 140 lbs, you should be aiming to eat about 98–140 grams of protein a day. Keep in mind that a chicken breast that is the size of the palm of your hand is approximately 20–25 grams of protein, and one egg is 6 grams of protein. Therefore, you should absolutely be eating protein with every meal and if you can't get enough of it with the three meals you eat, you may have to add in protein shakes or high protein snacks like lunch meat turkey roll ups (3–4 slices of turkey wrapped around a few pieces of lettuce with a bit of mustard or mayo depending on your liking).

Furthermore, breakfast will always be an important meal for you and you should make sure it's high in protein. Beyond helping to meet your required protein needs, a high-protein breakfast will also help set your energy level, blood sugar, and metabolism for the day and should keep you fuller longer. I like to start my day with a high-protein shake and a couple of eggs or a few links of chicken sausage. I aim for around 35–40 grams of protein at that meal.

Clients and patients often ask me about the protein powder I use in my shakes and how it compares to collagen powder. It's a very good question, and here's my answer. Collagen powder is excellent for hair, skin, teeth, and gut health. It's also supportive of ligaments and other soft tissues. But when it comes to a quality protein source, collagen does not have a full amino acid profile, so it's known as an incomplete protein and should not be relied upon for building muscle. Therefore, if you want to supplement your protein intake with a powder, make sure it's a complete protein powder—animal, whey, or plant based. Then you can add collagen powder on top of that to reap the extra benefits.

Beyond increasing your protein intake, round out your daily eating with as many healthy vegetables and fruits (preferably organic) as you like, and small portions of healthy fat like extra virgin olive oil, avocado, grass-fed ghee, and nuts. Focus on getting the majority of your carbohydrates from fruits and starchy vegetables like potatoes, sweet potatoes, a variety of squashes, and rice. At meal or snack time, strive to eat your protein first as it will begin to fill you up and prevent you from subsequently overindulging in carbohydrates and fats.

Implementing these guidelines into your daily eating with a focus on eating whole foods that are minimally processed can help you live a more vibrant next chapter of life and provide you with the sustainable energy you need to cultivate more purpose in your life after kids. Notably, if you commit to eating more protein, you will find that you are fuller and not in need of eating so many carb-heavy and sugary foods that lead to weight gain, blood sugar imbalance, fatigue, and inflammation in the body.

One last thing before we move on: Even the healthiest of eaters may find that their body is still lacking nutritionally because of stress, difficulty breaking down and absorbing food, and lack of minerals and vitamins in our food due to poor soil quality. Therefore, supplementation may become necessary, especially as we age. For a full list of beneficial supplements for women in midlife, refer here www.lifeafterkids.com/book.

Detox

Unfortunately, we can eat a healthy diet and focus on moving our body daily, but if we don't practice gentle detoxification from time to time, environmental toxins can build up in our system and damage our health and longevity regardless of our diet. To be clear, toxins can be found in the air we breathe, the food we eat, the clothes we wear, and even our household and body products.

While I don't want to add more stress to your life by worrying about the chemicals that you're being exposed to each day, I do need to make you aware of the toxic exposure to your body so you understand why an occasional detox is so important. Similarly, I don't want to overwhelm you with an in-depth detox protocol that is difficult to implement in your daily life—if it becomes too hard to do or it feels like a chore, it will become stressful, and you're likely not to do it at all! So let me highlight a few very simple things you can do a couple of times a week in order to cleanse your body of toxins.

Probably the easiest and most affordable thing that you can do to detox is to sweat at least 3–4 times a week, because every time your body sweats, it releases a buildup of systemic toxins. Twenty to 30 minutes is all you need and you can get a good sweat going by taking a hot Epsom salt bath (added bonus, the salt will help you detox further), or you can sweat during your workout.

If you have trouble sweating while you work out, try wearing a long sleeve shirt and or a sweatshirt, and if you exercise at home as I do, you can use a space heater in your exercise area to get the surrounding temperature conducive for a good old-fashioned sweat. Saunas are also a great way to sweat and thus detox, and saunas happen to be very beneficial for cardiovascular health as well as stress management. There are several companies that sell one- and two-person saunas that can be purchased for and used in your home. These in-home saunas can be pricey, so if they aren't in your budget, consider using a sauna at your local gym or at one of many med spas that seem to be popping up more regularly. Again, this could also be a great way to meet people and make new connections. As a side note, while hot tubs can be very relaxing and aid in reducing muscle tension, I would not recommend using them for detoxing purposes because, in most cases, there is a certain amount of chemical exposure due to the sanitization of the hot water.

You can go a little deeper in your detox with supplements like liposomal glutathione, which can aid your body in its own detoxing, and activated charcoal, which helps to pull toxins out of your digestive tract. Activated charcoal is so powerful that it must be taken on an empty stomach and completely away from medications/supplements because it will pull all the good nutrients right out of your system along with the bad.

One key thing to remember when you are gently detoxing for a day is you MUST stay hydrated. Because you'll be sweating, thus losing fluids and because you want to be sure you don't get constipated when taking activated charcoal, it is imperative that you drink enough water throughout the day.

The key to detoxing is being able to move toxins out of your body, first by sweating but also by moving your bowels. You must be going to the bathroom at least one time a day and fully evacuate to ensure proper movement of toxic waste products out of your system. If you don't regularly poop once a day, you may need to take a magnesium supplement (200–400 mg) and/or begin taking a potent spore-based probiotic, as well as eating fermented foods. For more on these supplements and fermented foods go to www .lifeafterkids.com/book.

Hormone Balancing for the Win

It's important to note that your liver is your body's primary organ for detoxing, and if you have a buildup of toxins in your body, your liver can become congested, making it difficult to do its job. This can create a whole host of problems in your body, not the least of which is hormone imbalance, since your liver is also responsible for removing excess hormones from your body.

It goes without saying that after the age of 40, hormones can make a woman feel miserable due to hot flashes, night sweats, moodiness, lack of sleep, headaches, excessive bleeding, and more. Hormone changes coupled with feeling stuck or lost because our kids are grown and leaving home is precisely why Dr. Lynne and I often refer to this phase of life as the perfect storm. Not only are balanced hormones important for our emotional health and well-being, but when our hormones are balanced, we have better bone density, healthier skin, improved sleep, faster metabolism, higher energy, and clearer thinking. As an added bonus, balanced hormones provide us with better cardiovascular health. For more information, check out the book written by Mary Claire Haver, MD, *The New Menopause: Navigating Your Path through Hormonal Change with Purpose, Power, and Facts*

I could write an entire book on balancing hormones, but because I only have this section for the discussion, let me touch on the main points to get you started and then I'll point you to other informative resources so you can take a deeper dive. Here's the most important thing that I believe you need to know about balancing your hormones:

> *Stress is one of the factors that creates hormone imbalance in your body, and this is important because you have the ability to manage your stress levels!*

When you go through menopause, your ovaries begin to slow down and lower their production of sex hormones like estrogen and progesterone. But your body still needs these hormones, so instead of being produced by the ovaries, your adrenal glands take over. Your adrenal glands are two walnut size glands that sit on top of both of your kidneys and, besides producing precursors for your sex hormones after menopause, they are also your stress-handling glands and they secrete cortisol and epinephrine.

Now imagine for a second what might happen if you're in a period of change and transition, fighting to maintain control of your life as it once was. You're struggling to let go of the past. And you're questioning who you are and what you want to do with life, while losing the battle with daily stress management. (I'm pretty sure I just described just about every mom entering into or already in an empty nest.) Do you think it's possible that your adrenal glands could become tired and focused more on stress manage-ment, stress hormones, and survival than on the production of sex hormones that help you through menopause? Spoiler alert! That's exactly what can happen. And on top of that, if your blood sugar is all over the place due to eating and lifestyle habits, your adrenal glands will try to balance it with cortisol production. Once again, the focus of the adrenal glands has shifted away from menopausal help to put out more immediate fires.

Allow me to sum this up in simple, concise terms: If you are struggling with menopausal hormonal imbalance to the point that it's affecting your physical and emotional health and you're looking for a natural approach, the two best, easiest, and most affordable things to do are as follows:

- Get laser focused on managing your stress (see Chapter 4).
- Make appropriate changes to your diet (i.e. more protein—it's a building block for your hormones, don't forget!—and less sugar) to balance your blood sugar.

Couple these two things with a healthier liver due to occa-sional light detoxing strategies, and you have a recipe for kicking major menopausal butt! That being said, perhaps you're in a situa-tion where you've had enough and you need more intense and targeted help. If that's you, go here www.lifeafterkids.com/book for more information on hormone healthy supplements, foods, and books we recommend.

Choosing a Healthier and More Purposeful Life Beyond Motherhood

Whatever approach you choose to take with menopause, I hope by now you see how important hormone health specifically and physical health in general is to you being able to fully thrive in midlife and pursue your passions and purpose beyond motherhood. The key here is that you must have enough energy and mental clarity, i.e., brain power, to put your all into pursuing a new purpose after your kids are raised.

Too many amazing moms are floundering in this phase of life feeling anxious, sad, and lonely, and they're blaming the way they feel solely on their kids growing up and leaving home, all the while believing there is no end in sight because their kids aren't coming back home. Though that may be the case, please understand that the foods you eat, your body movement (or lack thereof), your toxic load, and menopause are significant pieces to the thriving in life after kids puzzle.

Recall how important controlling the controllables are for overall happiness as well as emotional health and well-being in this phase of life. When it comes to our physical health and its relation to our happiness and well-being, we need to focus on the controllables once again. The good news is so many things are under our control when it comes to our longevity. We may not be able to control that we're aging, but we do have control over how well we age.

You have a choice. You get to decide. Do you want to grow old vivaciously with energy, spunk, and mental fortitude, being a great example to your grown kids while actively engaging with grandkids? Or will you take the path of least resistance, normalizing frequent aches and pains, lack of energy, brain fog, and gradual loss of independence as your body wears out, lacking the energy needed to pursue more purpose, never mind keeping up with your grandkids.

As for Dr. Lynne and I, we choose daily to do whatever it takes to keep ourselves healthy, well, and independent for as long as possible, and we know without a doubt that the attention and care we give to our physical health keeps us emotionally grounded, far less anxious, and far more focused, allowing us to fully engage with our older kids, our husband, friends, and our life after kids community, while relentlessly pursuing all of our hopes and dreams. I hope you'll join me on the road less traveled, the sometimes seemingly harder path that leads to a healthier and more purposeful life beyond motherhood.

Chapter 7

Beauty in Life Beyond Motherhood

By Dr. Brooke

What does beauty mean to you? That's s a loaded question, especially since we're part of a culture that has body-shamed and age-shamed women for so long that many of us do everything possible to look more youthful than we are. It's as if we're on a constant expedition to find the fountain of youth and, thus, deny our age. Is it just me or do you also encounter times when you stare at your reflection in the mirror and are taken aback by what you see?

Sometimes, it's like I'm not sure who that woman looking back at me is as if overnight I went from being a youthful twentysomething to being almost 50 years old. Where did those lines around my eyes come from? Is that more gray hair I see? And don't get me started on the forehead wrinkles that my esthetician so lovingly calls expression and laugh lines. Please! I don't know what could have possibly been so funny!

But let's get back to the question at hand. What does beauty mean to you? The Merriam-Webster Dictionary defines it as the quality or group of qualities in a person or thing that gives pleasure to the senses or mind. Pause for a moment and take that in. Because if this, in fact, is the true definition of beauty, then you and I need to get busy letting go of what social media, Hollywood, and the world at large tells us beauty is.

The dictionary definition of beauty does not say that beauty is thin, beauty is youthful and without wrinkles, beauty is long flowing hair without a touch of gray, or beauty is perky breasts or legs without cellulite. According to the dictionary, there is no one way for a person or thing to be beautiful. Instead, beauty is something that brings pleasure to the senses. It would seem then that beauty is relative. Beauty is in fact a perception, and indeed it is in the eyes of the beholder.

What's more, the above definition states that beauty brings pleasure to the mind. Being that we're wrapping up a section on building resilience with emotional balance, physical health, and mental fortitude, it seems as though now is the right time to have a discussion on something that brings pleasure to the mind, and that is beauty.

In this chapter, I want to discuss with you three specific areas of beauty along with their relevance for thriving in life beyond motherhood. These areas are *physical appearance, personal space,* and *the world around you.* I submit to you that all three of these areas of your life hold their own beauty and if you are intentional about cultivating and noticing their beauty, you will not only "give pleasure to your senses and mind," but you will also add more fulfillment to this phase of your life.

You Are Beautiful and You Need to Believe It

As previously discussed, Life after Kids is the perfect storm and our feelings of upheaval and overwhelm in this transitory phase of life are deeper and more complicated than our kids growing up and leaving home. In this phase of life, we're struggling with the status of our nest and our identity shift from being a full-time mother. We've also got our hormones raging as we enter menopause. And on top of that, we're grappling with our age/mortality and the changes in our physical appearance. It's a trifecta of struggles.

When you consider your physical appearance, my biggest hope is that you do it based on what feels right and looks best to you instead of what other women or society at large says. Further, I encourage you not to judge other women based on the way they look or what they choose to do with their appearance. Honestly, there is nothing more beautiful than a woman who feels comfortable in her own skin and confident about the way she looks. The things that make us different are the very things that make us special, and our differences should be celebrated.

Tackling the somewhat sensitive topic of physical appearance in midlife can be a bit tricky especially because we all have different ideas of what beauty at our age looks like. And there's no denying that advancements in procedures done in med spas and by plastic surgeons to slow or reverse the physical appearance of the aging process has significantly changed the landscape of the way a woman ages. With each day that passes, it feels increasingly harder to be a woman in her 40s, 50s, and beyond in a world where the ideal for what middle-aged should look is nearly impossible to obtain.

Somewhere along the way we seem to have lost the ability to accept the image looking back at us in the mirror and, if not love what we see, at least like it. In my own life, there have been many moments where I've gazed critically at my reflection in the mirror. On the mornings I have darker circles or extra puff under my eyes from a night of poor sleep or a day of eating that was subpar, I find it more difficult to believe that I am, in fact, resilient, lively, and vibrant. If I'm being brutally honest, on those days, I have trouble focusing on finding new purpose and creating change in my life because I can't seem to get past my age and the signs of it written all over my face.

Ladies, finding new purpose in our life now that the kids are grown is hard enough without self-sabotaging and distracting ourselves by things as frivolous as the way we look and how we are aging. Sometimes, we really can be our own worst enemy. And equating our self-worth with how we feel about our physical appearance is just plain ridiculous.

What would life look like if we set all the noise of the world aside? What would life look like if we stopped comparing ourselves to the way other women our age look? What would our life look like if we chose to get up every morning and smile at our reflection in the mirror? What if we got more comfortable in our own skin, accepting and embracing the aging process instead of fighting it. What if we began to fall in love with every part of our body, even our fine lines, stretch marks, and loose skin?

I do wholeheartedly believe that every woman should feel empowered to age the way she feels is best for and most beautiful to her, and we should hold space and have grace for all of our differences. But perhaps it's time to flip the script. Maybe we could all use a mindset shift.

Remember earlier when I said we should let go of the things we can't control and instead focus on what we can control? Well, it applies here, too. Because any feeble attempt that we make to stop the aging process is not going to reverse the clock or make us any younger than we are. And just as we must come to terms with our kids growing up so we can focus on our purpose and living a more fulfilling life, we also have to come to grips with and let go of our age.

Instead, let's focus on what we can control, which is our mindset. Let's talk about how we can all be more accepting of ourselves, the way we look, and the aging process. Let's remember that our wrinkles and fine lines are from time spent outdoors enjoying the sunshine and from years of laughter with our family and friends. Let's recall that our stretch marks are from carrying and birthing our beautiful children, making every imperfection and all the loose skin worth it. Above all, let's remind ourselves that aging is a luxury that so many people never get to have, and that the value we bring to the world is so much greater and more worthwhile than our outer appearance.

A Little Lip Gloss Goes a Long Way

None of us are aging in reverse, so one of the best things we can do to feel comfortable, confident, and beautiful in our own skin is to accept our age and accentuate the beauty that we already have instead of wasting so much energy and time trying to change it or make it better according to the world's standards. (For more tips on aging vibrantly and naturally, get our "Ageless Beauty Guide" at www.lifeafterkids.com/book.)

That being said, accepting our age and our physicality doesn't mean we should do nothing with our appearance and just "let ourselves go" altogether. I don't know about you, but when I feel good about my appearance and feel more put together, I feel better emotionally, and I am more productive. And doing simple things like getting showered, dressed, and putting on a little bit of lip gloss or tinted lip balm even on days you don't feel like it can do wonders for your emotional health. If nothing else, starting your day by giving your physical appearance some attention is a step toward keeping you emotionally grounded and focused on making the most of the day.

It's a small way to feel good about yourself and to execute what little control you have over the aging process. In the midst of the seemingly rapid change and transition of life beyond motherhood, having a sense of (even if it's small) and control of your world is important. Even the smallest of actions you take through the course of your day, like putting on an outfit you feel good in, can go a long way.

Now don't get me wrong; I enjoy a good day in my pajamas a few times a year just like anybody else, especially if it's a cold and cozy day over holiday break or I'm a little under the weather. Sometimes, it's necessary to take a personal day to rest and regroup.

But if those days are becoming more and more frequent, it's probably time to make a change even if you don't necessarily feel like it. Besides, haven't you also been in a situation where you stayed in your PJs because it was the holiday or a rainy, windy Saturday? You were determined to relax on the couch watching movies or binging a series on Netflix only to feel sluggish and worse at the end of your day.

Sometimes, even on the days you don't feel like it, you have to act the way you want to feel. Do whatever makes you feel better about your appearance. Take that shower. Apply a little lip gloss. Put on a favorite outfit. When you take these simple steps toward feeling beautiful, you may be surprised at how your mood or view of the day shifts.

Skin Care Routine for the Win

Similarly, simple things like skin care routines are not only great for your skin and accentuating your beauty, but don't discount that they can also help with your mindset as well because they are a form of self-care and self-love.

A little self-love and care to your appearance at the start of your day is just as important at the end of your day. Taking time for a skin care routine in the evening helps me unwind. I love the way a clean face feels and massaging cool, lightly scented moisturizer into my skin is relaxing while triggering my brain that it's time to prepare for a restful sleep.

Right before going to sleep, I like to apply a heavy dose of cocoa butter balm to my lips just because it feels so luxurious. In the morning, splashing cold water on my face and preparing it for the day with various products energizes me and gets me ready for what's ahead. The skin on your face is delicate, and it needs to be treated well especially because you present it to the world every day. And remember, the more radiant your face, the more radiant you'll feel.

Air Out Your Closet

As important as cultivating beauty in your appearance is to productivity and emotional balance, cultivating beauty in your personal space is every bit as necessary for thriving in this new phase of life. And cleaning out your bedroom closet and drawers while refreshing your wardrobe is an amazingly cathartic exercise that is a motivational symbol for letting go of the past and stepping into your bright and beautiful future.

Clothing and style can be tricky at this age because we often find ourselves in the gap of not feeling good about ourselves in clothes that are for a younger crowd while also not wanting to dress too old for our age. Fortunately for us, in today's world, we have so many options for style and shopping at our fingertips, with more and more middle-aged women stepping outside the over 40 and 50 fashion box, rocking their age and dressing to accentuate the beautiful female body in all of its shapes and sizes.

In summary, make a habit of getting dressed every day. Don't stay in your PJs and refrain from throwing on sweatpants and a bulky sweatshirt with your hair in a messy bun. Yes, some days are good for relaxing in sweats, but that should not be the norm. Instead, consider stepping outside of your comfort zone, and take some time to go through your closet, getting rid of things that no longer serve you and that you don't love. While you're at it, fill your closet with comfortable clothes you feel pretty and confident in.

Declutter Your Personal Space, Declutter Your Mind

Cleaning and organizing the rest of your home and closets has the same effect, if not more so. Understand that your immediate environment has a direct correlation with your mindset and productivity. If your living space is cluttered and messy, your mind is likely to be cluttered, and therefore, your productivity can suffer. In this phase of life, with so many of us longing for more focus and less brain-fog, any simple thing you can do to declutter your brain is a win!

Remember the words of Tony Robbins, "How you do anything is how you do everything." I've seen this play out in my own life as I cleaned out all of my closets, storage spaces, and entire home in preparation for a move to a new house. I cannot begin to describe how freeing it was to get rid of things that no longer served me or my family but that I'd been holding on to for years. Don't get me wrong: It was emotional especially going through my kids' old art, school work, and family photos, but it was well worth it.

When the process was done, I felt lighter and so ready to take on my future. Sometimes, to free up your mind and heart to new ideas, new purpose, and new passions, you have to start by freeing up your home and personal space. Letting go of things from your family's past doesn't make you any less of a mom, and it doesn't minimize all of the amazing years you spent raising your kids. But it is okay and healthy to let go of the past and move forward in new ways. Cleaning and organizing your home is one practical step in the direction towards re-creating your life now that your kids are grown.

Cultivate Beauty in Your Home

Similar to personal appearance, finding beauty in your personal space (home environment) will help you feel more emotionally balanced. So, take some time to do a few updates to your home if you haven't already. Perhaps you choose a new paint color for the walls or you change up your artwork, move your furniture around, or even buy some new pieces. So you don't get overwhelmed, pick one room in your home, preferably one you spend a significant amount of time in, like your kitchen, family room, or even bedroom, and start there.

If you don't have a large budget for redecorating, take heart because even smaller things like new throw pillows, blankets, or a new lamp can make a big difference, especially if you've already completed the task of decluttering, cleaning, and organizing. One of my favorite ways to maintain a positive mindset in my home is with plaques and artwork that contain my favorite inspirational quotes and scriptures.

I even have our family core values (Dr. Lynne spoke about these in Chapter 3) on three large plaques that I had customized, hanging in our entryway. Just be sure that if you're bringing in something new, you let go of something you already have so you don't over-clutter your home and, therefore, your mind!

Beauty Really Is All Around

Let's close this chapter by talking for a moment about the importance of finding beauty in the world around us. You might be wondering how this could possibly apply to thriving in life beyond motherhood. It's a good question. So, let me expand upon the topic to give you a simple and powerful way to live a more fulfilling life.

This phase of life can feel like a race against time. Most of us are busy creating a new chapter and adjusting to the change in our family dynamics. With the hopes of making the most of our time and living a meaningful and vibrant life, we're setting goals, dreaming big, nurturing our relationship with our older kids, taking risks, trying new things, and stepping out of our comfort zone. But in the midst of what could be described as midlife chaos, it's important to also pause from time to time and take notice of the simple beauties in life.

For example, when is the last time you got up early enough to see the sunrise or took a walk at sunset to view the radiant colors in the sky? Have you made time to go to a museum and ponder thought-provoking artwork? Do you pause to smell the sweet fragrance of the flowers in your garden? How about taking a hike or scenic walk to be awe inspired by the beauty of nature? Or take a trip to experience the beauty of various cultures and landscapes. Maybe you need to pause more often to give your spouse or loved-one a peck on the cheek or even spend a moment or two thinking about the beauty of your child's smile.

Whether it be the sunrise or the sunset, a stunning piece of art work, a song that gives goosebumps, travel, the feel of your beloved pet's fur on your hand, a smile from your child, or even better, a hug, these simple pleasures remind us of how beautiful life really is. They evoke in us feelings of immense gratitude for the life we are already living. They teach us not to take ourselves, our lives, or our age too seriously and they remind us of what's important and truly meaningful in life beyond motherhood.

Have you seen the movie, *Love Actually*? It's one of my favorite holiday movies. It begins in Heathrow airport with family, friends, spouses, and loved ones hugging each other after travel. Hugh Grant is the narrator and the scene begins with him saying, "Whenever I get gloomy with the state of the world I think of the arrivals gate at Heathrow airport." He ends the scene saying, "I have a sneaking suspicion that if you look for it, you'll find that love actually is all around." In the same manner, I believe that when you're feeling down about your life after kids, take time to cultivate beauty in yourself and in your personal space. Pause to enjoy and appreciate beauty in the world around you. Then you'll find that beauty really is all around. And you'll find that your life, my friend, is actually more meaningful and fulfilling than you imagined.

Part III

COMMUNITY AND FRIENDSHIPS

Chapter 8

You Can't Do It Alone

By Dr. Lynne

The Difficulty of Meeting New Friends: It's Not Just You

When we first decided to post on our Life after Kids social media pages about friendships in this phase of life, we did so because it's an authentic pain point for us, too. Dr. Brooke and I had each other, but because we don't live close geographically speaking, we were both craving quality friendships with women who shared our values and interests that also live in our communities.

The response to this topic was WILD! Though we can't seem to collectively agree on politics, our religion, or our parenting styles, it seems the majority of our community overwhelmingly agrees that with our kids leaving, we are more prone to loneliness and that good friendships are more important than ever.

There are three fundamental problems to point out when it comes to making new friends in this stage of life: access, time, and comfort. Acknowledging these problems will better help us to find the appropriate solutions.

Problem #1: Access

The first reason it's more difficult for you to make friends is simply because in general there are fewer new people encountered in this phase of life. Building lasting friendships is a numbers game— you've got to meet enough new people to find the alarmingly few that will match your values, interests, and situational circumstances (like agreeable schedules or distance). If you attended a post-secondary college, those years may have been your lifetime peak of new friend-making. Everyone on campus was in the same boat, eager to meet others and form new connections and groups. That emphasis we placed on our social life tends to extend for quite a few years, throughout our 20s and early 30s, more or less, until family priorities take over.

After that, due to the increased energy demands it requires to raise a family, most people narrow their social focus significantly to a far smaller circle. Some good news—there is often frequent exposure to new people through kids' activities and school. These kinds of shared experiences with your kids' friends' parents can even be powerful enough to bond together people who don't have much else in common. Because of this, it's a unique and almost passive period of friend-making, similar to that of your own school years. When your kids age out, stop activities, or they grow up and leave the home, that pipeline subsequently dries up. Typically, after that time, you will have to exert more effort to find new people to become friends with.

Problem #2: Time

The second problem in making new friendships in midlife is evident in the consistent and quantitative time investment new friendships require. It takes abundant time and frequent exposure to each other in order for a budding friendship to develop. When I think about the length of time and work I've invested into my friendship with Dr. Brooke it feels overwhelming to think about starting that process from the beginning with someone new. Most of you still have many other responsibilities and family needs competing for your time. Between your work and running the home, modern life is simply busier and more demanding than ever.

Emerging friendships require you to dedicate chunks of time that you may not have readily available. Even if you're committed to making the time to prioritize new friendships, you are just 50% of the equation. You'll need an equally committed friend who's also willing to carve out some time to invest in the relationship, in order for the bond to flourish.

Problem #3: Comfort

The third difficulty in making new friends in this phase of life is a nuanced problem that is significant nonetheless. By this point in our lives, a lot has happened both good and bad that has shaped us into the people we are today. You've lived a lot of life and you represent a cumulative history that gets harder and harder to download for someone new, the older you get. Naturally, it is harder to feel close to someone who hasn't shared in some of these prominent life experiences with you. Therefore, many women tend to lean on their well-established friendships for support in lieu of finding new friends even if those friendships have gradually become damaging or are no longer adequately meeting their needs.

The familiarity and the strength of the bonds that are formed from shared life experiences can magnetically pull you back into a comfortable albeit dysfunctional relationship. For new friendships to form, a few ingredients must be cultivated: curiosity, openness, patience, and excitement for learning another's life story. Each of these ingredients can compensate for a lack of shared bonding and familiarity, but it will definitely take some intentionality to overcome the tendency to retreat back to what's most familiar.

Making Friends Is Good for Your Health

Collectively, it's extremely healthy to keep an open mindset and foster excitement for meeting new people and gaining new friends. It's actually a matter of our survival to do so! Social isolation and loneliness are serious risk factors for your health. A group at Stanford has reported that having strong and secure relationships could increase the length of your life by as much as 50%.[7,8]

Even though this is true for every one of us, Dr. Brooke and I know that meeting new people and making friends comes easier to some of you than it does for others. Whether or not meeting new people and making new connections feels natural for you, the research is very clear: Every human benefits from maintaining broad and deep social connections as they age.

In Chapter 2, I referred to the landmark research study by Harvard scientists that took place over an 85 year span.[1] The researchers began this study in 1938 with the primary aim to investigate exactly which factors cause people to flourish. They began with 724 participants with boys from disadvantaged and troubled families in Boston as well as a number of privileged Harvard undergraduates. The study eventually incorporated the spouses of the original men and later nearly 1,300 descendants of that initial group.

The researchers periodically interviewed the participants, had them complete questionnaires, and collected biometric information related to their physical health. The participants were studied through a myriad of life's major transitions—falling in and out of relationships, finding success and failure at their jobs, and becoming parents. It's the longest running in-depth study on human life to date, and the primary result is both simple and deeply profound. The results revealed that the most important, unequivocal indicator of health and happiness throughout our lifetime is the presence of *positive relationships*. According to this research, positive relationships make us happier and healthier. Period.

At first, I had many hesitations about tackling the complicated topic of friendship in this book. However, I came to realize that I have a lot of experience, both good and bad, to share on this subject. I am pretty blessed to have some amazing friendships with incredible women even though it's taken me my whole life to learn how to attract and retain these types of friends. I know firsthand what works and what doesn't. I'm going to share my "scar tissue" in hopes that you will sidestep those mistakes I've made and use the same lessons I've learned to feel incredibly connected and supported in your friendships.

Friendship Mistakes

If you are someone who feels that you are already fairly adept at making friends, count yourself as extremely blessed. Easily forging deep connections and winning new people over are a couple of additional examples of the hidden talents we spoke about in Chapter 3.[10] If you haven't yet stopped to recognize how cool and special these traits are, here is your invitation to do so now. Use your natural talents to foster new connections for yourself and take it a step further by lending a hand to someone who seems to struggle in this area. Practice widening your circle and allow those to come in who might need extra time to warm up.

For those of you who have shared with us that you need help, we've got you. We see you and we understand what that feels like to be lonely or feel like you're missing out. Because it's just plain harder to make and keep friends for the reasons we explained above, prepare yourself to work harder than you may think to find your tribe and subsequently nurture those relationships that will enrich and expand your life. I usually appreciate knowing the scope of the challenge that lies ahead so I'm better prepared to take it on. I hope you find this disclosure beneficial as well.

Although the friendship-making process can be arduous and lengthy at times, feeling more at ease and being more effective in the presence of new people can absolutely get easier for you overnight. Here are a few important things to avoid to find the friends you're seeking and some ways to better communicate more efficiently and effectively when you do.

Friendship Mistake #1: Misreading Your Social Energy Tank

Energy is everything. Without it, we can't pursue any of our heart's desires and we certainly can't be the best kind of friend possible. Remember those needs we described in Chapter 2? If you recall, the first tier refers to your basic physical needs. Having sufficient energy is a huge piece of what enables you to meet that tier.

If you're a beginner to our work, we gently remind you to build the foundation laid out for you by Dr. Brooke in Chapter 6 first. We are firm believers in the concept of like attracts like especially when it comes to energy and values. If you're looking for vibrant and healthy women to engage with, first increase your vibrancy and health by taking the necessary actions to improve your diet and fitness. It's not about looking like a supermodel; instead, it's about increasing your energy from its source. As you reconnect to yourself again, consider also the capacity of your social battery—what gives you a natural boost and what leaves you feeling drained.

Introvert vs. Extrovert

Growing up, I would have traded anything to be like my older sister. If you grew up in the shadow of an older sibling, maybe you can relate. Paula was five years older than I was and much cooler than I thought I was at the time. This wasn't a fair shake because I was comparing my 13-year-old awkward middle schooler self to a high school senior and a brunette Farrah Fawcett look-alike at the time.

Looks aside, the thing that I really envied about Paula was her natural charm and easy-going nature with people. It seemed that she had oodles of friends and she never felt compelled to stay home with her nose in a good book on a Friday night as I did. And the way she charmed new people whom she would meet at a store or getting on the bus was clearly a natural talent. I was in awe.

All of these years later, I'm still a card-carrying member of the Introverted society. As it is with your unique abilities, your default as an introvert or extrovert is hard-wired from a very young age. Everyone's individual degree of introversion/extroversion lands somewhere on a dynamic sliding scale. You can slide up or down a few degrees toward or away from the midline but it's very rare and next to impossible to flip from one end of the spectrum to the other. Your wiring and programming never change that dramatically even with major life changes and upheavals. For this reason alone, it makes sense to stop wishing to be like someone else and start loving yourself for the special person that you are.

I realize that I've held an embellished belief in the meaning of the terms introvert/extrovert over the years. Frankly, I've misconstrued both definitions while also underplaying the importance of knowing where I fall on that spectrum. I've spent years in denial, trying my hardest NOT to be introverted, not really liking what I *thought* that meant for myself.

Looking back, this 100% prevented me from making and building authentic connections with friends along the way. I'm sharing it with you in case you need to get it straight, too. Mistakenly, I believed that an introverted person was brain and book smart but not necessarily people smart and was often awkward around others or even socially inept. I also believed that extroverts were gregarious, outwardly communicative people lacking intellectual depth that could never sense when to stop talking.

A few years ago, I read Susan Cain's book titled *Quiet: The Power of Introverts in a World That Can't Stop Talking.*[14] It was her book that revealed that my previous definition of introverts and extroverts was way off base. Susan says this: "Introverts are simply people who recharge their batteries by being alone. Extroverts need to recharge their batteries when they haven't socialized enough." This clarified definition allowed me to shed some restrictions and limiting beliefs that I had about myself.

News flash: You can be smart AND inwardly focused AND be well-liked, funny, and socially confident at the same time. On the other side of the coin, if you're socially proficient you can also be intellectual and have depth and layers to your personality. Labels placed on us can sometimes be helpful, and other times, they can harm us. This is one instance when a label dangerously prevented me from seeing my whole self.

The most significant reason we should know where we land on the introversion/extroversion scale is because it allows us to properly care for ourselves and alleviate drain on our resources. Knowing a surefire way to increase your emotional energy stores is an important part of caring for yourself. When you take better care of yourself, you can take better care of others, including your family and your friends. That's a missing link for many women. If you're not hyper-aware of how you recharge and what you need to feel refilled you may be draining your battery too low, too often.

Dr. Brooke is extroverted. She and I have the good fortune to spend several weekends a year traveling together, sometimes with mutual friends, as couples, or with our families. Because we don't live near one another, I used to feel the demand to spend as much time with her as I could in the time we were given. I would often push myself to the limit and come home feeling drained and grumpy.

Now on these special occasions, I usually duck away here and there throughout the weekend to take time to recharge. During a recent four-day seminar filled with plenty of "extroverting" dinners out, I joyfully passed on Saturday night's group dinner. I kissed my extroverted husband and sent him out the door to meet our friends while I ordered room service and then proceeded to sleep for 12 hours. The old me would have soldiered on and pushed myself to go out, but once there I would have been low energy, short, and inwardly resentful.

As you can imagine that mood doesn't lend itself well to the development of meaningful connections. Now that I've correctly gauged my social energy tank, I'm more likely to embrace the

JOMO (joy of missing out) over the FOMO (fear of missing out) when my stores run low.

Be accepting of your need to recharge often and acknowledge how this might be different from your husband, your kids, your best friend, even your own Mother. Be prepared to communicate proactively that you may need to step away to recharge your batteries but that doesn't take away from how much you adore them and cherish your time together. This is a crucial course of action for introverts who wish to maintain their relationships while still taking the time they need to be alone.

If you're extroverted with an introverted spouse and/or friends, be ready to explain how recharged you feel by spending time in the presence of others. It's necessary for your loved ones to accept that it isn't that you prefer other people over spending time with them, it's simply a matter of energy procurement for you—it's how you're wired. When you're feeling drained, your course of action can be to get out of your house and have time with other people in order to refill your energy tank.

Friendship Mistake #2: Comparing Yourself to Others

In the long list of social mistakes to be made, comparing yourself to others is perhaps the worst offense of them all. You can always find someone doing better or worse than you in whatever measurement you're using. Therefore, comparing yourself to someone else is completely ineffective when it comes to helping you feel better about yourself.

Comparison is the root of jealousy and unwelcome competition, both of which are so destructive to our friendships. As I mentioned, I have some truly amazing women friends. Now that I reflect on it, I've managed to surround myself with women who inspire me to be better because of how committed they are to show up as their own best selves.

All of my best friends are accomplished, kind, funny, and beautiful. It would be easy for me to look at them and feel less than.

I'm not going to pretend that I haven't gone there and spent more time than I'd like to admit in that comparison danger zone. Here's the thing: When I indulge in that behavior, I don't feel good. It's like eating a greasy cheeseburger—once it passes your lips you instantly regret it.

When you focus on what your personality lacks and not on what you do well, you're ironically overlooking the many special traits you possess that stimulates others to envy you! Whatever your comparison is tied to, whether it be material things, such as expensive homes or clothing or if you think she's skinnier or more likeable than you, remember this. It's absolute torture and a total waste of time to go there. Don't do that to yourself and don't do that to your friend.

When you notice yourself heading into the comparison zone, reframe the situation by refocusing yourself on how unique you are and feel pride for your many fantastic gifts instead. Accept that you are both on the same journey; you may just be at different points along the way. Many of you have lectured your children on this very thing—it's time to own your specialness and focus on winning your own game now.

Friendship Mistake #3: Mismatching your Personality Type with Others

If you haven't taken our Enneagram quiz to find your Enneagram type, it's a good time to revisit that now. Understanding your Enneagram type is a subtle but effective strategy for improving friendships. Dr. Brooke is an Enneagram Type 6, and I am a Type 1. Enneagram Type 6s, aka The Loyalists, are like Labrador Retrievers as friends. By their nature, they are fiercely loyal and sincere. There are so many good things about each of the Enneagram types, and as her friend who adores her, I look for opportunities to validate those good qualities in her.

On the other hand, Type 6s can also be skeptical and mistrusting at times. This used to get under my skin, truth be told, until I was better able to see where it was stemming from. It was a big a-ha moment and a pivotal turning point in our friendship.

Three years into our business partnership, I'm certain we would not have been successful in keeping the friendship intact and flourishing without knowing these specific details about each other. Now if she openly doubts what I have to say, I don't take it as a personal attack. As a Type 1, my tendency when someone doubts me is to take it personally, for instance, doesn't she know how hard I'm trying to get things right and perfect over here?!

I now use my knowledge of the Enneagram to develop a deeper understanding of all of my close friends. You don't have to be an Enneagram expert to use this information in your relationships to your advantage. You just have to know the basics, be willing to ask questions, and stay curious enough to dig beneath the surface. We recommend getting your friends together for a fun night with some good wine and food. After everyone has settled in, have them take the Enneagram quiz (or better yet, send out an email with the link beforehand).

Once people have an idea of their type, they will take their turn talking about their type as it relates to their life. There's an elevated chance that the evening will end with you all feeling closer and better understood by one another than before. To make it easier for you to plan and execute a Girls Night In in the way we've described, we've made a PDF with step-by-step instructions. You can download your copy at www.lifeafterkids.com/book.

Friendship Mistake #4: Not Communicating Productively

Let me point to a powerful ripple effect as I tie this together. Honest communication has been a key to prevent hurt and feelings of rejection in most of my friendships. I've had to confront some tough situations with good friends along the way but almost every time I've been brave and caring enough to address it head on, the situation has improved and the relationship itself has become stronger.

Be proactive and share some of the things that you learned in this chapter with a friend. If your girlfriends don't know that you need time with them to recharge (for the extroverts) or without (for the introverts), how will they honestly know you and where they stand in your life? If you can't be vulnerable with them and at times admit that you have self-doubt or question certain things about yourself, they won't know where your triggers and insecurities lie. You may have to be the one who initiates these conversations by asking questions of your friends about themselves that help you go deeper.

Here are some starter questions to stimulate more in-depth conversations:

- Do you need more or less friend time now that your kids are out of the house?
- What are you most proud of about yourself?
- What has been the hardest part of raising your kids? The easiest?
- What is your love language?
- Do you feel you are introverted or extroverted? Why?
- How do you like to be comforted when you are sad or upset?
- What do you hope life looks like five years from now?

It's a great time to have these types of conversations because our needs are changing and our friendships are becoming a higher priority. Opening the door to more intimate topics related to our true selves can lead to more satisfying and deeper connections. When you know your friend better, you can more readily give them the gift of your trust and full acceptance. At the core, this is how world class friendships develop.

Chapter 9

Finding Your Tribe

By Dr. Lynne

Back to Basics: Friends 101

I have four precious grandkids ranging in ages from two to eight years old. We recently attended the first soccer game of the season for six-year-old Jovie. There isn't really anything much cuter than a pack of six year-olds swarming a soccer ball up and down the soccer field like a busy cluster of bees. The best part isn't how they interact on the field—it's their interactions off the field that fascinate me.

Even though the team was assembled for the very first time just moments earlier, there were already excited conversations taking place, impromptu hugs, and a couple of girls bouncing up and down while giggling out loud together. Six-year-olds have instantaneous friend-making down pat. Here's the play-by-play. Walk up to someone, tell them your name, ask them a question or two, end the entire encounter with a cartwheel, and then repeat. Well done kiddos, well done.

News flash: Making new friends is pretty much the same now as adults as when you were a kid minus the cartwheel. The reason little kids make it look so easy is because they have yet to experience the negative downside of putting themselves out there socially. As grown women, we are usually keenly aware that making the first move in a new friendship might lead to a rejection. Most women will do almost anything to avoid that. The conundrum is we must assume that risk to have the desired outcome—a possible new friend.

On the other hand, you could sit around waiting for someone else to make the first move. I'm convinced that the reason so many women are struggling in this area is because they prefer to take a passive role and wait for others to come to them. The tragedy is this: Everyone is drowning in the same lonely sea and few are willing to throw a life preserver by making the first move.

Picture yourself in the following scenario. There's a possible new friend from a yoga class or someone you've seen walking the neighborhood that you'd like to initiate a conversation with. When the opportunity strikes, remind yourself of the following two things so you can muster enough courage to make a move. There are so many women in your community who are craving new friendships, too—the odds are in your favor that you'll meet someone looking for a connection, too, so take the chance! Second, when putting yourself out there, never, and we mean never, hang your self-worth on the line. Some people will get you and some will not.

The fear of rejection has held me back more in life than I care to admit. In my 50s, I've finally embraced that I'm not everyone's cup of tea, and likewise, I don't want to be everyone's best friend either. This makes me feel more resilient and more likely to happily get on with life with less emotional backlash when a rejection does occur.

The mantra I use to help me deal with a possible self-rejection is this: Some people will like me, some won't, so who cares, and who's next? Remember we told you making friendships is a numbers game? It's my experience that from 10 personal encounters, you'll be lucky to have two or three emerging friendships. Another two or three will be total duds, with the remaining four to six connections classified as somewhere in the middle.

The Rule of Threes

Practically speaking, I've found it helpful to adopt the rule of threes in regard to my relationships. The rule of threes says you can characterize the companions in your life as one of the following: three-hour friends, three-day friends, or three-week friends. Each of these three friend types serves a purpose in our life, but it's important to know that the friend types should not be measured against each other or held to the same standards. Each layer represents a different potential and capacity for connection. Imagine having to fill a vase with different sizes of river rocks, and pretend that this vase represents the amount of time you have to give to friends. The best strategy will always be to fill your vase first with the large boulders (three-week friends), followed by the medium size rocks (three-day friends) and finally the small pebbles that fill in the gaps (three-hour friends). Even though the three-week friends will take up much of our time, the other types can also play an important role in our lives. Combined, all of these friendships create a rich and multi-layered social network.

The goal is to have as many three-week friends as time allows but the higher likelihood is that you'll have many more three-minute and three-hour friends readily available to you. Be sure to invest time and energy into these friend layers as well. Some of these friendships could develop into a deeper layer of connection if they were to be cultivated more often.

Often, it comes down to shared values. We tend to more effortlessly tolerate those people who share a similar set of values and approach to life. That said and given our current political climate, I want to remind you that you benefit from a challenge to your way of thinking and those people in our life who live and think differently than us can help us grow. If we ONLY spend time with women who think the same, we tend to narrow our mindset. I encourage you to remember that your values and beliefs become strengthened through opportunities to engage in healthy and respectful debate. Therefore, there's immense value in interacting with women who think differently about politics, life choices, and religion even though they may not make your innermost circle. As moms, women, citizens, and humans, we share so much in common, it's a shame when our relative differences completely overshadow all that we can agree on.

Friendship is a two-way street. Many of you have expressed frustration over having to give more than you feel is being returned from a friend. In the Bible, Paul tells us that Jesus said, "It is more blessed to give than to receive." That's difficult to argue with although it's admittedly harder to put into practice. Whenever there is an uneven exchange of time, effort, or concern between two friends, there should be no delay in addressing it. I regularly see social media posts containing the message to swiftly walk away from "toxic" relationships, effectively cutting certain people out of your life without hesitation or pause. While I agree some friendships eventually run their course, have we become too quick and eager to wipe the slate clean and abandon our friendships? Instead, is there not something more satisfying found by taking greater pains to understand their point of view and to learn more before you cut and run?

When women tell us they have a shortage of good friends, I think what they're actually saying is they have too few friends who take the time to get to know them on a deeper level and for whom they feel seen, valued, and understood. If this is true for you, I believe there is one clear path forward. *Be the friend you wish to have.* In other words, be willing to do for others what you ask for in return. When it comes to building authentic friendships, you are only limited by what you are willing to give. If you have a tendency to put walls up, you will likely be met with walls in return.

I'm not saying that you shouldn't be cautious of friends who don't bring out the best in you or who secretly wish you will fail so they can be happier about themselves. There are times when friends need to be demoted to a lower rank. But before you go that far, openly and honestly communicate how you feel. Let's do more communicating and less ghosting. Most people purposefully avoid hard conversations because they don't want to hurt feelings. We ignore the problem, rationalize it and/or try to downplay how much we feel hurt because we're afraid of confrontation or we're afraid if we speak our feelings others won't like it. So, we avoid the truth. Following this trajectory, you either lose your self-respect by not speaking up or the relationship reaches maximum tension. This type of heightened emotional state between two friends typically leads to a powder keg explosion—usually sparked by a small, seemingly innocent transgression that indicates there's a deeper, unaddressed issue to blame.

If you opt to stay in that place of "like" in lieu of confronting and sharing your true feelings, you risk never moving towards greater intimacy, connection, and love. It may be uncomfortable to talk about the heart of a conflict, but clearing the air and speaking openly will usually leave you better off both emotionally and energetically.

The Four Types of Moms

The formula for being a great friend is similar to being a great parent or mentor. In addition to being accepting, available, and respectful of your feelings, a great friend inspires you to be your best. It's much easier to do this for a friend when you have a greater understanding of what they're capable of.

In relationships, *opposites often attract*. We are often drawn to other people because of a subconscious awareness they possess a personality that's complementary to ours because of our differences. However, after the initial "honeymoon" period is over, ironically those same differences we were initially attracted to often become a major source of friction.

As we do life together, we commonly fail to account for our respective coping strategies in managing life's daily stresses. This scenario can seriously derail a friendship. When we have better language to understand one another, it lends to us becoming more forgiving and appreciative with each other especially during hard times when we need it the most.

The Four Mom Types is our subjective interpretation of the proprietary work of Gallup, Inc., who originally identified four domains aiming to equip individuals with specific language to describe the power and edge of their strengths. You can find your Mom type by taking our quiz at www.lifeafterkids.com.

Disclaimer: Your Mom type result is not intended to confirm or indicate your domain of Strength or your leadership style as determined by the CliftonStrengths Assessment. It is strongly advised that you take that assessment at https://store.gallup.com/h/en-us for the most accurate result.[4]

Mom Type: Remarkable Relators

If you're a Remarkable Relator, your superpower is rooted in your ability to make connections with ease. Your friends think of you as the glue that binds and brings the group together. You're a true pro when it comes to seeing others, being likeable, and making others feel important and included.

The speed to which you can make a personal connection with others is envy-able! Maybe you're not "flashy" or wanting to lead the pack like some of your friends, but your good-natured personality is extraordinarily attractive, and you effortlessly put others at ease. You're a Mom who understands that it's the people in your life that are most important, and at the heart of everything, relationships are the currency that makes your world go around.

You effortlessly navigate your relationships with empathy and graciousness.

Never forget how highly valued your special ability is especially to those who are wired differently than you are. Others will easily be attracted to your easy-going nature and want to work alongside you because you usually make working more fun and you remind us to prioritize the people in the equation over the results.

Some people might misread your harmonious and amiable nature as weak or lacking authority. But you know the truth: There is massive power in having a high relational IQ. Of note, many Remarkable Relators truly thrive in their caretaking roles and are quick to pitch in and give of themselves especially when it's for the people they love. No matter what you do, choose opportunities to work with, for, and alongside people. You're likely to fade working or volunteering from home without others to interact with or spending too much time alone, period.

Friendships may come easily to you, but you would likely benefit from more self-awareness when it comes to setting boundaries. Because of your genuine love of people, you might have trouble saying no.

How to Be a Better Friend as a Remarkable Relator

You're the friend who doesn't hesitate to reach out when someone is struggling or has experienced a loss. Whether or not that's been confirmed, I'm confident your friends love that about you. Take that a step further and take the initiative to get your friends together for a night out or weekend away. You probably get plenty of invites due to your easy-going nature, your friends will appreciate you stepping up to plan and take charge once in a while.

Mom Type: Diligent Doers

If you're a Diligent Doer, your superpower is in GSD—"Getting Stuff Done!" You're a pro when it comes to the "how" and "when" of moving the needle on a house or work project or in general, taking ideas and making them reality. Completing tasks and taking action is your natural inclination.

You're the person people come to when they know a job must get done. You might not even be the leader or in charge, but others seem to know you will reliably carry your pursuits across the finish line. You are no nonsense and usually ready to get to work.

Some people might misunderstand your drive to be productive and think you care more about completing tasks than you do people. But you know the truth: Doing IS caring. You show that you care by DOING things for the ones you love.

You bring action and the ability to see anything you do through to completion!

It would be a mistake to lose sight of how highly valued this special ability you possess is especially to those who are different from you. Others usually benefit from your "get 'er done" spirit in working alongside you.

Friendships don't always come easily to you. Relationship-building takes precious time, time you usually prefer to be using to get things done!

How to Be a Better Friend as a Diligent Doer

You're the type of friend that steps in to take action when a friend is struggling. You may not know what direction to take, but you'll be boots on the ground once the work is started. Challenge yourself one step further and turn your relationship-building into part of your to-do list. Schedule time for reach outs and get-togethers in your planner well in advance.

Don't think of friendship time as idle time or time wasted; reframe it instead as another "important project" to work on and prioritize connection time as part of this objective. Planning a party and pulling off the details won't be too hard for you, so rely on your skills in this area to help with boosting your social calendar.

Mom Type: Magnificent Motivators

If you're a Magnificent Motivator, your superpower is embedded in taking charge, speaking up, and making sure others are heard. You're a pro when it comes to motivating and inspiring others to get on board whatever ship you are sailing.

You may not be a celebrity or a famous person, but you still manage to influence most people you come into contact with in some way. You're a mom who understands that persuasion is an art, and only a select few are gifted with it.

Some people may misinterpret your charismatic nature as fake or feel threatened by your rock-solid self-assurance. You innately know that influence is power. You show how much you care by being the voice for those you care about especially if they cannot do so easily for themselves.

You have an uncanny ability to convince others of your point of view.

Followers come more easily to you than friendships. You can be a lone wolf unless you're actively searching for others that can match you in presence and charisma.

Remind yourself often of how highly valued this special ability is especially to those who are not the same as you. Others are generally attracted to your magnetic presence and want to work with you.

How to Be a Better Friend as a Magnificent Motivator

You're the type of friend who is usually the voice for your friendships. You may not be great at the details and you may have trouble following through on what you say you will do, but your excellent communication style can make up for a lot. Remind yourself that actions speak louder than words, and the more time you take to plan the better especially when it comes to your friends.

Mom Type: Awesome Analyzer

As an Awesome Analyzer, your superpower is absorbing and analyzing information to inform better decisions. You're a pro when it comes to gathering and using information to expand others' thinking for what is possible.

The speed at which your brain works is enviable! Even if you don't care for the term "book smart" (although chances are good that you are), your thinking is undoubtedly innovative and creative. You're a mom who understands that slowing down and taking some time to consider the best strategy before proceeding forward will save ample time in the long run.

Some may underestimate your analytical nature as "overthinking" and incorrectly label you as uninterested or detached. But the truth is the thoughts and ideas you have circulating in that brain of yours is just more entertaining for you than small talk with other people. Conversations that require thought and debate are usually stimulating, however. You can be animated and engaging with others as long as you've had sufficient time to entertain your thoughts or visions for the future on your own.

You keep everyone focused on what could be and inspire new ideas with your creative style of thinking!

Friendships may not come easy; nevertheless, you crave connections with people who can match wits with you. Ironically, you are often drawn to those whose social skills seem to be their primary talent.

Never forget how highly valued this special ability is especially to those who are simply wired differently than you. Others will be attracted to your visionary nature and will want to work with you to help make your ideas reality.

How to Be a Better Friend as an Awesome Analyzer

You're the kind of friend who gives great advice because you've spent time looking at the problem from all angles. You may not be great at showing affection and you may sometimes be your own best friend, but you're generally an extremely understanding and forgiving friend because you can see the circumstances from a wide lens and a strategic standpoint. Challenge yourself to turn those thoughts into words of affirmations for the people you care about. If it's easier to write your thoughts instead of speaking them, start by doing that. Just don't take for granted that the people you love and admire know how you feel about them.

Practical How-to's for Making Friends

Friendship Tip: Commit to Making the First Move

My father, Brian, passed away several years ago. It was not sudden, however it was still a shocking and deeply sorrowful time for our family. We held a long Irish wake for him, and there was a constant stream of people who came to pay their respects. His funeral took place a few days later, and despite a terrible Canadian blizzard, hundreds of people braved the weather to honor my Dad.

A few days later, when my family gathered to share our individual experiences from the wake and funeral, a couple of interesting patterns emerged. We collectively realized our Dad dubbed most everyone with a personalized, playful nickname, and so many people privately shared with us how endearing that simple act was. They didn't know he did that for everyone, but most said they would always remember him for it.

The second pattern was also striking. His beloved close friends, of which he had many, reminded us of how systematically he approached his friendships. Every day he would use the right breast pocket of his signature button-up shirt to carry his cordless phone everywhere he went. At the wake, his friends spoke to us about how he'd call them, sometimes daily, but no less than once a week. They were genuine and effusive in their appreciation of this regular contact because he made them feel important and valued by methodically reaching out.

This was an important realization at the time, and I think his friends would agree we can all take notes from Brian Ryan on how to build and maintain friendships. His example reminds me to commit to making the first move even if at first it's not reciprocated, pay attention to the small details, and regularly take the time to reach out to the people you care about.

Friendship Tip: Put Yourself in the Right Places

The more exposure you have to new people, the more likely you will make a friend. Another tip is this: *Look for places where you'll find plenty of other people who are also looking to meet others.*

Think community gyms, community centers, country clubs, volunteer organizations, church gatherings, and sports leagues as concrete examples. If you have a sincere interest in something and there is a group setting that revolves around that particular activity, you will have at least one shared interest with everyone you meet there. Running clubs, hobby clubs, political action committees, and birdwatching groups are other examples that come to mind.

Friendship Tip: Make It a Memorable Meeting

All new friendships start with an initial conversation, which is arguably the hardest and scariest part. It takes some chutzpah to walk up to new people and start talking to them in hopes of turning that stranger into a friend. In these first interactions, most people start and end with overly familiar conversation starters such as "What do you do?" "How are you?" and/or "Where are you from?" However, to fan the friendship flame, there has to be enough interest peaked by both parties in those first meetings. Try working in a few more stimulating conversation starters in addition to the basics when meeting a brand new friend. The following are some examples to remember:

- Tell me something you're excited about lately?
- What's a new skill you're trying to learn or a hobby you're excited about?
- Have you done something really fun this week?
- What's the best thing that happened to you this week?
- Do you have any fun plans for your weekend?

Notice these questions are designed to elicit a positive response. When asked one of these questions exactly the way they're written, the brain will automatically search for an appropriate positive response resulting in an unexpected mood boost to some degree.

There's some time-saving benefit built into this tip as well. Their response to your questions can help you quickly decide if you should put further energy into pursuing a friendship with them, saving you time if it's not a match.

Friendship Tip: If You're Scared, Don't Do It Alone

Another suggestion to increase your chances for success at first meetings is to recruit a friend who thrives in situations with new people to be your wing woman. There are plenty of women who feel completely at ease in crowds of new people, and they are actually fairly easy to identify. These are the people who talk to strangers wherever they go. They can't help themselves from engaging in small talk in the elevator or making friends with the person they're seated next to on an airplane. They're a specialized type of extrovert who become energized by the opportunity to talk to someone new.

If you have some trepidation when it comes to meeting new people and you're lucky enough to have one of these friends, recruit her to attend new social situations with you. You'll both benefit, you by having a supportive ally in those first meetings and her through a greater exposure to new people.

Friendship Tip: In a Sea of New Faces, Be Ready to Throw a Lifeline

Recently on the podcast, Dr. Brooke shared a story about attending a New Parent Mixer at her son's new high school. She went alone, and she was late, therefore, she found herself walking into a room full of people already engaged in many small group conversations. Picture it—with no initial luck in finding a familiar face, she strolled to the bar and stood there alone pretending to do important work on her phone. She did that until she was rescued by a small group of women who stepped up to introduce themselves upon noticing her standing there alone.

First off, can we applaud these women for making that first move so graciously? After some small talk, Dr. Brooke also did something worthy of applause. Instead of coolly trying to play it off, she was transparent and thanked them for making the first move.

She straightforwardly admitted she didn't know a single soul before they had approached her. Right after that, someone made a joke about not knowing what to do with your hands whenever that happens, everyone laughed, and the ice was effectively broken. What could have been an awkward social moment ironically provided an opportunity for a bonding moment. Another tip here: Frank honesty can be a fantastic ice-breaker. Don't be afraid to just tell it like it is.

Friendship Tip: There's No Match for a Face-to-Face Connection

With a little effort, you'll eventually find some potential new friendships that you must now cultivate. Friendships are built and solidified by spending time together. One of my closest friends, Camilla, says "There's nothing like an energy exchange between two humans that only comes from being together under the same roof!" Although staying connected through texts and phone calls is a productive and important way to stay connected between in-person meet-ups, it's no match for physical togetherness, laughing together, and sharing the same experiences in the same moment.

Having regular check-ins to look forward to keeps the friendship alive and strong. My time-saving suggestion to bring friends together is to *plan a low-stress get-together for several friends at once.* Emphasis on low stress. The Barefoot Contessa Ina Garten says "The best parties are the ones where the host is having as much fun as the guests." You should be free to enjoy your guests and not running around doing pick up, serving a complicated meal, or trying to keep your guests on a schedule.

Friendship Tip: Invest Time Daily to Cultivate Stronger and Longer Lasting Friendships

Thankfully, maintaining and fostering our relationships regularly takes far less energy than finding and developing new ones. To develop the trust and intimacy you've built so far, you will need to *consistently invest your time to keeping those connections strong. The following suggestions might appear obvious at first but we suggest taking inventory of what you're already doing to stay connected with friends and then identify at least one of these easy-to-implement ways you can use to bump up your efforts:*

- *Acknowledge them with a text or note a few times each week:* It doesn't have to be a hand-written note, but when you see or hear something that reminds you of a friend send a quick text and let your friend know. You may readily underestimate how endearing something quick and easy like this can be. This is the perfect opportunity to subtly let your friends know that you are here for them and you care! If you don't seize the opportunities to tell her, how will she know how you feel?

- *Send personalized memes, quotes, or links:* I love the recent trend of sharing Instagram video reels with good friends. As your friendship grows, a personalized meme or video let's her know you see and understand her special traits. This works like glue to strengthen your bond. I'm usually taken a little off guard by how meaningful and personal it feels to have a friend reach out to me that way. It helps me feel more connected to her, and because it takes so little time to do, I've deemed it worth a mention.

- *Choose an appropriate communication method with your friend's preferences in mind:* I've recently made some new friends in a group and one of the women in particular is intriguing to me and someone whom I felt inclined to get to know better. I've observed firsthand her gift of communication (she likes to talk and she's good at it). In lieu of sending a customary friendly text one morning, I picked up the phone and called her with a question. It extended into a longer conversation and since then she's also called me a couple of times. With our pervasive texting culture, we can easily forget that texting is no match for an actual conversation. Sometimes, you just need to pick up the phone and call your friend.

  However, don't be offended if this doesn't work at first—talking on the phone isn't for everyone. Whether it's via phone, FaceTime, Zoom, email, written note, or text, choose different methods for different friends and consistently reach out to the people you care about or care to know more about. Dr. Brooke actually sets a daily reminder in her phone to reach out, which I think is a great way to prioritize your friends amidst the busyness of your days.

- *Support her personal growth or interests:* Ask a friend to volunteer with you or pick up a new hobby or sport together. As your kids become grown, you're likely both in a phase of rediscovery. Ask her more questions about her interests, goals, and passions. Having someone willing to jump in on new ventures with you is obviously a huge perk of friendships right now.

Friendship Tip: Look to Your Role Models

If you feel like you could use a little extra help in the friendship department, remember that success leaves clues. Look to the people in your life who seem to have an abundance of quality relationships in their life. Study them and you'll probably find that they spend a good amount of focus and energy cultivating and strengthening their connections.

You Need Me and I Need You

It bears repeating, no matter what you do or how you go about it, you need people to live a happy and fulfilled life. Many of you are introverts and you may be convinced that your own company is sufficient on most days. Look, we know that relationships can be messy and difficult at times. Even the healthiest and most evolved relationships still carry a risk. The more open and vulnerable you allow yourself to be, the greater the chance of being disappointed or let down by a friend.

Maybe you're not afraid to get hurt. Maybe you simply get busy doing life and you don't take the time to let those people who enrich your life know what they mean to you so that friend-ships can further develop. Wherever you stand, when it comes to your friendships, it's undeniable that your friendships are the dif-ference maker for your happiness and longevity. Finding ways to improve and increase your communication and having more understanding and grace for them during the bumpy times is so worth your efforts in the end.

The sooner you start investing time in your relationships and the more frequently you engage, the easier the whole process of friendship-building will become for you. Give yourself permission to make mistakes and in so doing, remember that your self-worth is never at stake if a friendship rejection occurs. Accepting others for who they are and allowing them to more fully be themselves in your company is the greatest gift you can give. With any luck, you'll enjoy this gift in return. When you get this right, I truly believe you'll feel as if you are winning in life.

Part IV

FULFILLMENT IN YOUR LIFE AFTER KIDS

Chapter 10

Risky Behavior Isn't Just for Teenagers

By Dr. Brooke

"No pressure and no hard feelings," she said. "I've been talking about it for several years and this year I am climbing that mountain whether you join me or not. I am prepared to do it by myself if I have to." Dr. Lynne wholeheartedly meant every word as she related to me early on in 2021 that one of her goals was to hike a 14er, which is a mountain that is 14,000 feet in elevation.

I knew she was serious, not only because I know her well enough after all these years to read her body language and her tone of voice but also because she had been talking about hiking a 14er for several years and this was the first time she ever threatened to do it by herself. If I'm being honest, I wasn't super keen on hiking a 14er; this was not my dream. It was Lynne's, and frankly I was just lukewarm.

But Lynne and I are each other's ride or die, and I knew she was mentally preparing to hike that mountain by herself. So, I thought it was in both of our best interests to do it with her. We then roped our good friend Sarah into taking on the adventure with us. It's funny how sometimes in life, your friend's goal becomes your goal as well.

I wish I could tell you the hike in Colorado that began on a cold, clear, and dark October morning was amazing and I was well prepared, taking time to stop and breathe in the environment around me, while enjoying every moment. The reality was, I spent almost all 10 hours of that hike wishing I was anywhere but on that mountain as I puffed fresh oxygen from my hand held pump in a feeble attempt to acclimate to the altitude.

The hike was grueling. It seemed to be never-ending especially because we had to stop regularly to catch our breath and gain our footing. And if that wasn't enough, when we got to the summit, a snow storm complete with thunder and lightning rolled in. PSA: Standing on a 14,000-foot slab of granite in the middle of the clouds is not exactly where you want to be during a thunderstorm. Needless to say, we all but ran down that mountain, adrenaline fueling our flight back to tree level where we would be out of immediate danger even though we'd still have miles to walk before reaching the parking lot and the safety of our car.

As I opened the door to the rental car that afternoon, sitting down for the first time in about 10 hours, I wasn't sure whether to laugh or cry or scream. Honestly though, I was too delirious with exhaustion to do anything but kick my hiking boots off and grab something to eat from my backpack. The three of us sat quietly in the car as we refueled, rehydrated, caught our breath, and just generally wrapped our brain around what we had overcome and accomplished. We barely said anything on our long drive back to the hotel, coming to grips with the fact that we not only scaled a 14,000-foot mountain, survived a snow and thunderstorm, but more importantly, and perhaps the biggest feat of all—we overcame every negative thought in our head that told us we were not capable of reaching the summit.

You know the voice—the one we all hear from time to time that says, "You're too old," "You're not capable," "You're not strong enough," "Your time has passed," "Who do you think you are," and of course, "Why even bother?"

It's Not Comfort and Safety That We Need

For me at least, it's precisely when these voices rear their ugly heads that I know it's time to tell them to shut the heck up and march headlong into the exact thing I'm reluctant to do or even scared of. And if you want to live a more fulfilling life now that your kids are grown, you'll start telling those voices to get lost and begin to push yourself out of your comfort zone too because pushing yourself and taking more risks is exactly where the fulfillment happens and the fun begins.

Ironically, when Lynne and I talk in the Life after Kids community or on our podcast about pushing ourselves harder and seeking continuous growth, some moms push back, saying they've worked hard all their life and they're ready for a rest. They ask, "When is it finally time to kick back a little and just enjoy being?" And I get it; there is a time and place for rest and being content with what is especially because we've spent most of our adult life parenting and running on steam. I agree that rest, regrouping, and landing in a post-child raising comfort zone does feel good in many ways and may be necessary for at least some period of time. But if you stay there too long, it will never afford you the purposeful and meaningful life that you're seeking.

I'll admit that staying where you're comfortable is reassuring and easy, and sometimes I just downright crave easy. But let me pose a question to you that I hope you'll seriously consider:

Is relaxing and staying in your comfort zone, seeking peace and status quo, what will really make you happy in life beyond those rigorous years of full-time mothering, or are you choosing the comfort zone because you're listening to and believing those crummy voices whispering incapabilities and lies in your ear?

I bet if you take some time to ponder this question, you'll find that you excuse living in your comfort zone by telling yourself these stories: "You deserve it after all these years," or "Taking it easy is what every woman wants in this phase of life," or "The path to happiness is the path of least resistance and work, and it's high time you had a rest." But what's really behind the story you're telling yourself is fear. Fear that you'll fail and fear that those voices are right. Besides, if you try and you do fail, will you tell yourself, "What will everybody else think of me?"

Get ready because I'm just about to answer all those questions with a cliché that's probably going to annoy you, but here it is anyway *You won't ever know until you try*. And trying almost always involves risks.

The Benefits of Taking Risks

It's on the other side of taking risks that the good stuff of life resides. When you make yourself uncomfortable by taking a risk, you're taking a step toward self-growth and creating more meaning in your life. In fact, as you work toward your goals, chasing down your dreams in this phase of life, you may wonder from time to time if these goals and dreams big enough, and how do I know if I should be reaching for more to really step into my purpose?

Here's the answer: You know when your goals and aspirations are big enough because they're a little bit, if not a lot, scary, and if you aren't working toward something that's at least a little scary, then you might be selling yourself short. Remind yourself that you are a strong and capable woman, and you were created for just a time such as this. You have gifts to give back to the world. Don't keep those gifts wrapped up tightly in the box of your comfort zone. Instead, start getting okay with being uncomfortable, so you can unpack your gifts and share them with the world. That's where you learn to love yourself more, gain more confidence, become more self-assured, and begin to realize that you are capable of so much more.

Self-Confidence

You'll recall from Chapter 6 that every time you push yourself through a hard workout you'd like to quit because you're sweaty, breathing heavy, and shaking, or just plain tired, you grow. And you don't just grow your muscles, you grow your capacity to believe in yourself and gain a deeper understanding of what you are actually capable of. You build confidence in yourself by pushing yourself, and that happens outside of the gym as well.

Remember also that affirmations have a positive effect on emotional balance and are very impactful for a more meaningful life after kids, but affirmations are only the first step. For example, one of my daily affirmations or mantras is "I am healthy, strong, and capable." The more times I remind myself, the more my brain believes it and I begin to own it. But you know what will get me to own my strength, capabilities, and worth far more quickly and concretely than saying things? It's doing them. And that's where risks come into play.

Let's use the example of public speaking. Say your goal is to get involved with a nonprofit organization that you are passionate about and one of the requirements is to speak at local community centers or churches to raise awareness around the cause. Likely you have some level of trepidation around public speaking as it is a very common fear. But if you really want to serve that organization and make a difference, you have to take the risk and get up on that stage.

And sure, you can prepare yourself by speaking daily affirmations and practicing what you'll say, but the best way to become a skilled speaker is to get in front of the room and do it, sweaty palms and all. The good news is that the first time you do something is when it's the hardest. After that, it gets a little easier every time. Suddenly, you'll start to see yourself as a public speaker. You'll have more self-confidence and you'll have an identity shift.

Identity Shift

Identity shifts happen to be another benefit of risk-taking. Who you think you are says a lot about what you will do in life.

For instance, if you're constantly telling yourself things like, "I don't make friends easily," and "It's just how I'm wired," or "it's easier to be alone," you'll begin to identify yourself as a shy, keep-to-yourself person. But as Dr. Lynne has discussed, research shows that connection and relationships are one of the keys to a happy, long, and vibrant life.

We should make friendships, and connection an important part of our life. But we'll have such a hard time making new friends if we believe we're shy, and we won't get over feeling shy just by telling ourselves we aren't or wishing we were different. If you want to get over your shyness and adopt a new identity, you have to push yourself out of your comfort zone. You have to take a risk like joining a book club or reaching out to a neighbor to go for a walk with you. It may feel scary, but once again, the more you do it, the easier it will become, and the sooner you'll shift your identity to being someone who makes friends easily and connects with people readily.

Life Lessons

Along with building self-confidence and shifting your identity, another benefit of taking risks is the life lessons you learn. And the good news is you'll learn something about life or yourself whether you succeed at the risk you've taken or if it's a colossal failure. If you take a risk and succeed, you'll learn that you are perhaps more capable than you gave yourself credit for and you'll have learned lessons that will prepare you for the next task at hand.

But let's say you take a risk and you don't succeed at what you were doing. Say, for example you decide to start a new business and after a year or so, you realize it's not going to work and you have to shut the business down. Well, and I'll say this as gently as possible: so what?! If nothing else, when you fail in this way, you'll learn that life goes on and that failure is not the end of the world. As you move on from the thing that didn't work out, you'll learn tenacity, perseverance, and resilience. These three things are muscles that don't get strong unless you fail or have a setback from time to time, and tenacity, perseverance, and resilience are necessary for living a more fulfilling and meaningful life.

Similarly, imagine you took a risk and began a new job only to realize that you didn't like it or you weren't good at it. This is actually not a failure; on the contrary, it's one of the biggest life lessons you can have because you learned about what you don't want to do with your life.

That's the funny thing about finding your purpose; sometimes, you have to learn what you don't want by taking a risk and trying something, and then having that something not work out before you actually stumble upon the very thing that lights you up. Besides, wouldn't you rather try something and know for sure one way or the other, rather than look back at your life down the road, wondering "what if"?

A Higher Purpose

Taking risks also enables us to leave our mark on the world and make it a better place. I'm going to get biblical here for a moment, please stay with me.

I want you to consider Moses for a moment. He is traditionally considered the author of the first five books of the Old Testament. This text relates that Moses was chosen by God to lead the Israelites out of slavery in Egypt into the wilderness that eventually led to the promised land. Moses could have easily stayed in his comfort zone in Egypt. As Pharaoh's daughter's adopted son, he could have lived a life of luxury in Egypt with very little work or risk. But instead, he chose to follow God's path for his life which was definitely not the easiest route. He not only took a huge risk by leaving behind his birth land and a significant amount of wealth, but he also had to face his fear of being incapable due to difficulty with his speech.

Moses not only took a risk to fulfill a higher purpose and leave his mark on the world, but he also had to overcome his innate fear of public speaking and trust that he could lead the Israelites even though every negative voice in his head was telling him he wasn't good enough. Moses chose to leave his comfort zone, step out in faith, and believe big for his life, and you can too.

Now maybe you aren't going to speak to God in a burning bush or etch something as historically important in stone as the Ten Commandments, but every act of fulfilling your purpose in this world, be it big or small, will allow you to touch the lives of other people and leave the world a tiny bit better than when you found it. Isn't that what we all really want at the end of the day?

Our Kids Learn from Our Risks

Our kids are watching everything we do. Every time we dream big and take a risk, stepping out of our comfort zone, we teach our kids to be brave and do the same in their own life. Remember, our kids learn far more from watching what we do than us telling them what to do. Do you want your grown kids to choose faith over fear in their own life? Do you want them to make the right but often harder choice in order to live a more purposeful and meaningful life? The best way you can ensure they do this is by doing it yourself.

When I dropped my middle son off at college for the first time, a four-hour plane ride away from home, he was nervous to say the least. The last night we spent together in the hotel room before he moved into his dorm, he related as much. My son stated he was worried about making new friends and going to social events as he is a bit of an introvert. And I advised him in this way, "Andrew," I said, "I'm not going to lie; it's going to be hard, but usually, the right path is the hard path, not the easier one. You could play it safe and keep to yourself, looking forward to when you come home again, or you could take a risk and put yourself out there, knowing that after the first time, every other time will be easier."

I went on to tell him, "Understand that you won't become your best self and gain the most out of life by staying where you feel the safest and the most comfortable. You'll grow the most and become all you were meant to be when you take risks and do things that feel just a little bit scary." As I sit here writing these words to you now, I hope that the words I spoke to Andrew several months ago were even more impactful because he not only heard me say them, but he's watched me live them.

When to Play It Safe, When to Take Risks, and How to Know the Difference

Without a doubt, risks are an important part of living a fulfilling life beyond motherhood, but there are times in your life when risks are not advisable and can actually cause more harm than good. Sometimes, it's more prudent to play it safe.

For example, if you're feeling nervous about investing a portion of your savings or retirement into an endeavor that you know little to almost nothing about, the nerves are probably there to keep you protected against losing money, and it's likely a good idea to stay where you are comfortable and not take that risk. Similarly, what if you were dreaming about selling your home and your belongings, moving into an RV and traveling the country? This type of a goal would feel scary to almost all of us. It's a big lifestyle change. But for some of us, it might be just the right amount of risk to take. So, how do you know the difference?

When you are considering a goal that is scary, or you are considering taking a risk in this phase of life, ask yourself these types of questions:

- Can I afford this?
- Am I comfortable with the sacrifices I'll have to make in order to make this happen?
- How will this affect my children and the rest of my family?
- Is my spouse on board, and if not, why?
- Have I asked advice from trusted friends or family members and what are their thoughts?

- If this doesn't work out, will it drastically change my life for the worse on the other side?
- Am I properly managing my stress and am I emotionally balanced and physically healthy enough to weather any stress or storm that comes along with this risk?
- Does this risk align with my core values and life vision?
- Is this a good match for my unique abilities and strengths?

Make no mistake, there are times in your life when you should jump right in and take the risk, but often, with bigger risks, you must lay the groundwork and ask the right questions to be certain that this risk, while big, is one worth taking and that the benefits outweigh any downside.

Once again, sometimes you don't know if you'll like something until you try it, but please be sure that if something does not work out, it won't wreck your life or leave you far worse off than when you started. In short, ask the question: Is this risk worth it and are you sure it's one that you are willing to take?

Here's where things get tricky because you must have enough discernment and self-awareness to know the difference between two types of fear:

1. Fear that is healthy and protective, keeping you safe from something you shouldn't do
2. Fear that will hold you back and is rooted in a lack of self-assuredness, lack of confidence, or concern about capability.

If you are wavering, it is often prudent to seek counsel and advice from a trusted confidant while also spending quiet time in self-reflection and prayer to be sure you are saying yes or no to taking a risk for the appropriate reasons.

Moreover, in a situation that you really can't seem to find clarity on whether to take the risk or not, it may be prudent to make a pros and cons list to help you make the right decision. Just be mindful that more often than not, risks are worth taking and your fear is likely due to you being uncertain about leaving your comfort zone. Remember, even if you fall short, you will have likely had a great learning experience and you will have built resilience and perseverance. Perhaps the best question you can ask yourself then, is, "What's the worst that could happen?"

Risks Don't Have to Be Big to Be Impactful

Remember that risk-taking looks different for different people because we're all wired differently. What pushes one mom out of her comfort zone and makes her palms a little bit sweaty might be a breeze for another mom. That doesn't make that risk any more or less valid for the person taking it.

So, when it comes to risks, don't compare the ways in which you are pushing yourself to anyone else around you. The only person you should be comparing yourself and your risks to is the person you were and the risks you took yesterday. Yes, there are big risks we can take in this phase of life, like hiking a 14,000-foot mountain for the first time, training for a marathon, starting a new business, selling your home and moving to a new area, or speaking on stage in front of a large group of people. But there are other seemingly smaller risks that can be taken, and while they may appear to the onlooker to be "small," they have no less of an impact. These are risks like calling an old friend you haven't talked to in years to reconnect and catch up, beginning your first ever weight training session, forgiving someone who has wronged you, deciding you are going to be your authentic self and not "bend to fit in," or getting a new hair style or make over. Any and all of these count. Maybe for you it's simply taking the time to smile and introduce yourself to somebody new.

No one else can live your life for you and nobody but you knows the boundaries of your comfort zone and what feels like "risky" behavior.

Make every effort to push yourself, to do the thing that feels just a little bit scary, and you will see your confidence grow and your bandwidth for pushing yourself and envisioning what you are actually capable of sky-rocket.

Ensuring You're Taking Risks with the Life after Kids Goals Framework

When re-creating your life after the kids are grown, you need strategic tools in place to make sure that the changes you seek for a more fulfilling life actually happen. Discussing its importance and saying you're going to do it isn't enough. Please know that it's okay to go at a pace that feels comfortable to you. You don't have to suddenly start jumping out of planes. You don't have to quit your job to begin a new venture or hike to the top of Mount Kilimanjaro. Similarly, you don't even have to commit to taking a risk every single day. (Although, at some point in time, you may build up to seeking to do one thing that feels uncomfortable daily.)

For now, let's just focus on picking two to three risky things that you can commit to doing over the course of a year. For me, this year, I committed to joining a fundraising group at my son's school. It was a risk for me because I'm already strapped for time so adding one more thing to my schedule felt uncomfortable, and I HATE asking people for money! The second risk was committing to making new friends and developing those relationships. Remember, I said that risks don't have to be big; they just have to push you out of your comfort zone for growth to occur.

To make risk-taking even more certain to happen in your life, write your risks for the year at the same time you plan your yearly goals. Along with everything else you are working on including but not limited to health, self-development, spirituality, and contribution, add two or three risks to the list.

I strongly encourage you to get the Life after Kids Goals Framework for this endeavor. On it, you will find a section for listing a few risks you're committed to taking. Remember, writing goals gives them a significantly higher likelihood of happening. Also, be sure to keep your Goals Framework in your planner or on your desk/work area so you can refer to all your goals and risk ideas often. You can get a downloadable version of the framework at www.lifeafterkids.com/book. Reminding yourself of your commitment to stepping out of your comfort zone by seeing them and saying them regularly will get you on the path to making them happen so you can live your best life after kids!

The Beauty of Taking Risks in Life Beyond Motherhood

Two days after I trekked that 14,000-foot mountain with Lynne, I was back on a plane headed home, tired and sore all over with achy feet. As the plane began its initial descent into Boston, I watched the GPS tracking of the plane on the small monitor in the back of the seat in front of me. Slowly, we were coming down in altitude: 35,000 feet, 28,000 feet, 25,000 feet, and so on. I will never forget the moment the monitor registered 14,000 feet, triggering me to look out the window of the plane to see in plain sight just how high I had climbed.

I gasped when I saw that we were still in the clouds, and I'm pretty sure my heart may have skipped a beat when I viewed the minute size of the land and buildings that could be seen through those clouds below. I think that's when what I had done really hit home. I had climbed on my own two feet, at the age of 45, so high that I was in the actual clouds. Boston, my home and starting point, would have been a town built of tiny Legos below me. And getting to that height didn't require technology, wings, an engine, or even a GPS. What it required was belief in myself, a friend who not only believed in me but could see all that we were capable of, and most of all it required will power and the willingness to push out of my comfort zone and take a risk.

There were times on that mountain that I struggled to catch my breath and other times I was certain that my legs were going to buckle underneath me. But even as my physical body wanted to give out and was telling me to quit, my mind took over, telling me to keep going. And because I kept going and pushed myself out of my comfort zone, I learned I was capable of far more than I ever dared to dream. Taking the risk of climbing that 14er quieted all those voices that say, "You can't," "You're not capable," "you're too old," "You'll never make it," and "You're not strong enough."

When those wheels finally touched down in my home city, I knew that I would be forever changed. That's the beauty of taking risks in your life beyond motherhood. You will learn resilience, tenacity, perseverance, and the ability to believe more fully in yourself and your capabilities. These are such precious and invaluable gifts. Please believe me when I tell you that if you want more from your life now that your kids are grown—more purpose, meaning, vibrancy, and fulfillment—then you have to put your fears aside and you have to commit to taking a step, big or small, out of your comfort zone. Because, sometimes, doing the scary thing is where the magic happens.

Chapter 11

Just Keep Growing

Dr. Lynne

Life Is Finally Getting Good . . . or Is It?

About four years before the pivotal conversation during our hike in New Hampshire when the idea of Life after Kids first material-ized, I spent a few years consistently feeling a sense of restlessness and boredom.

I was initially stumped as to why. We'd built a modest nest egg giving us a taste of more financial security than we'd ever had. Regular workouts were now on autopilot resulting in good energy levels throughout my days. In addition, the most rigorous and exhausting years of building our practice seemed to be behind us. My daughter, Lila, was a pre-teen and was fairly self-sufficient, allowing me extra time to devote to my own needs.

Balancing the moving parts of my life was taking far less effort than it once did. However, instead of basking in this reprieve from my chaotic young mothering days, I found myself bored and actively on the lookout for new fires to put out.

I spent about four years like that. Whenever something went wrong at home or at work, I'd huff and complain loudly about the inconvenience of it all, but at the same time, I also felt a little excitement bubbling up in those moments. Surely, I wasn't *enjoying* the fact that things were going wrong?

After many episodes consisting of me working diligently to calm things down only to have something else go wrong, my husband noticed a pattern and bravely called me out. I remember the knowing look he gave me that preceded his words. He sort of cocked his head and narrowed his eyes a little as if he was putting all the pieces together. I don't remember exactly what he said but it was something like—"I've been watching you run to the rescue of others too often; is it possible that you're feeding into some of these problems so you can have something to fix?"

My guns were immediately drawn. How dare he suggest that I was somehow contributing to these mishaps that kept happening! A younger version of me would have dug in, willing to go to battle, and die on that hill. But the older and wiser version of me knows very well that I married a smart man with my best interests in mind who does not have a previous track record of saying things purely to offend or anger me.

I also know that when a person has an intense reaction to something said about them, there's often an unpleasant kernel of truth in what was said that they're unwilling or reluctant to confront. Just because you don't like what you hear doesn't mean that it's not true. Our knee-jerk reaction is usually to blindly defend ourselves in lieu of objectively considering if there is any truth to the point made. In doing so, we forego an opportunity to learn and grow.

Truth time. I was a little excited with each new opportunity to spring to the rescue. As a result, I was not prioritizing enough time to better equip our leadership team, allowing for them to feel underutilized and stunted. I had reached a plateau in my personal learning and growth which had eventually led to boredom. As disruptive as it was, bouncing in and out of crisis mode was providing me with some much needed stimulation.

Embracing Relentless Growth

Growth is a top-tier need. It's not absolutely required for survival, however it is essential if you want to live an extraordinary life after kids.

The truth is, when you stop growing you start dying. If this sounds a little harsh, let me explain. If you're not actively growing, then technically you're staying the same. However, time and the natural process of aging ensures that nothing ever really stays the same. Because life is constantly moving forward, if you're not embracing a growth mindset to keep pace with the natural decline of age, then you will be falling behind. The further you fall behind, the more you decline. At that point, you will technically be aging faster than your years.

The most accessible way to grow is through the process of learning new subjects, skills, or creative pursuits. All of us have endless potential to learn; however, some of you have a higher than average predisposition for learning. In fact, it's one of the 34 unique talents identified by the Gallup organization in the CliftonStrengths Assessment. If you have some of these "superlearner" traits it can be a big advantage at this time in your life. Armed with a strong desire to learn, you may be more likely than your peers or spouse to engage in adult learning. You may not understand their lack of drive to learn or get frustrated when they don't share your learning excitement. This is another reminder that we're all crafted differently, and that no one way is the right way for everyone.

If you strongly agree with most of the following statements, you may be a Superlearner and possess a special propensity for adult learning:[10]

- You possess a *strong desire to learn ways to improve* in many different areas.
- You enjoy the process of learning as much or *more than the outcome of learning.*
- You more *frequently crave new opportunities* to learn than others around you.

- You may feel a desire to take on many learning experiences at once, not necessarily to get to mastery, but *mostly for the thrill and enjoyment of learning.*
- You have a tendency to focus on what you don't know versus what you do know, and varying degrees you have an *insatiable* need to know more.

When my husband and I first learned about our unique abilities, we discovered that I was a Superlearner. To solve any problem, I'd look for answers in a textbook or seminar whereas Mark preferred to jump in and figure things out through trial and error. I was resistant to fix anything until we had learned more. The result is I distrusted his hands-on approach and he felt stunted by my need to continuously study more prior to taking action.

Following a couple's life coaching session, we gained a better understanding of our respective problem-solving styles. Subsequently, we stopped judging each other for our differences and went to work on combining our styles. I would handle the initial research and root out two or three of the most promising solutions. Mark would then jump in to test each one to find the very best option. This synergy has outfitted us with a far more powerful approach to tackling life's problems than the previous method, which consisted of us relying on our individual respective styles.

I can't tell you how much this "superpower" has reinforced us throughout our marriage. It's exciting for me to know that there's always more to learn and understand about ourselves and the people we love.

As much as it is a strength, my insatiable need to learn has also created friction at times. I share my cautionary tale for other Superlearners to reflect on. An overeager student at times, I can get bored easily and ping pong between hobbies and new activities. My love of learning pursuits has been misunderstood at times and I've been asked some discouraging questions such as "Why are you spending so much time on that?" and "Will you be sticking to this?" This level of disdainful feedback subsequently resulted in feelings of guilt and fueled attempts to minimize my compulsion to learn new things.

My life drastically improved when I embraced that I'll always be drawn to learn new things though it may not appear to be practical or logical to others. I've adopted the following perspective: *I feel energized and alive when I engage in a variety of adult learning opportunities; therefore, it's vitally important to my well-being to find ways to learn as often as I can.* Fortunately, there are many free and low-cost ways to learn that also won't take up too much of your precious family time.

What happens if you don't necessarily feel a compelling desire to learn or you would not identify yourself as a Superlearner from the criteria we provided? Even if you're a proud creature of habit who finds comfort in following the same routines and doing the same things, you can still add in variety.

For example, if you're a faithful runner, try adding in a new route once a week or make the jump to swimming in the summer months only. In my observation, the people that crave the familiar and routine are not set in their ways as much as they thrive by having a standard framework to follow to keep things less complicated.

Keep the structure and experiment with the variables that you CAN change easily. For instance, assign one free hour of your week to do a new activity or just pick a new restaurant on your designated night to eat out. Change is a necessary element that can be easily absorbed inside of your well-planned life if you think creatively.

Daily Enrichment for Moms

In addition to your own personal growth, it's very important to act today to ensure your brain is healthy 20 years from now. What we do today determines our brain health in 10, 15, 20 years and beyond. Current statistics show that one in nine people age 65 and older will be diagnosed with Alzheimer's disease.[8] There are many factors that contribute to this condition, but the consensus is that if you can protect your brain from environmental toxins, maintain healthy blood glucose levels, and continue to fight cognitive decline by challenging and stimulating the brain in appropriate ways you mitigate your risk. Besides regular physical activity and having a healthy diet, mentally engaging activities are excellent for fighting the natural decline in brain health as you age.

With more free time, you can bet that I'll be at the front of a pasta-making class at my local Williams Sonoma or registering for French classes at the local community college after my youngest graduates this year.

However, if I wait for more free time before I start my practice of learning, I'll have a fraction of the brain health and personal growth that I could have if I found ways to bring some learning into a normal packed work/school week instead. Like exercising your body, if you wait until there's more time before you start working out, you're more likely to stop when life gets busy and that extra time is no longer available. Life will always be busy, so by fitting what's important into your busy schedule now, it can remain a priority even when life gets extra hectic.

Here are some practical, low-cost ways to exercise your brain daily:

- Download the *New York Times* games app. Challenge yourself with the Wordle™, Connections™, Spelling Bee™, and/or Mini Crossword™ puzzles each day.
- Register for the online platform MasterClass™. Engage in a course from a subject matter or celebrity expert. Choose from their large library of topics and switch from topic to topic when you get bored, guilt-free!
- Read something every day. Seems intuitive, but still worth mentioning. Some people hold off from reading books until they have time to sit for hours. Listening to audiobooks in the car is a great way to consume information on the go. Alternatively, if you commit to reading just five pages or

approximately 10–20 minutes a day, you will eventually read about nine average-sized books a year! Historical fiction and personal growth books are my go-tos for learning while being entertained at the same time.

- Perform your normal daily tasks in a brand new way. For instance, drive a new route to work or change the hand you normally use to brush your teeth or use your computer mouse with. These "switch-up" activities maintain existing neural connections in your brain and promote new ones to grow. Stimulating your brain this way has a similar effect that lifting weights does for our muscles.
- Treat conversations with strangers or friends as learning experiences. Ask more exploratory questions to learn more about their life. Fostering a heightened sense of curiosity about people and things can provide a constant stream of new and stimulating input for you.
- Pick a topic of the day and research it online.
- Block off a recurring time in your calendar solely for exploring your interests and learning pursuits. What gets scheduled, gets done. During that time, you can choose to fill that time with whatever feels most titillating to you that day or pick up where you left off in your last scheduled learning block.

You Can Slow Down Time

You need to do more than you've ever done in this phase of life to stay engaged and continue learning because it's so common to have less novel stimulation in your everyday life at this phase. You may have to work harder to get exposure to new things. The payoff is that with every learning experience, you create new memories and therefore a richer expression of your life.

As I get older, I have found myself getting more and more concerned with how fast each year seems to fly by. As it turns out, seeking more growth and having more novel learning experiences can actually help with this problem as well. *Inc.* magazine[11] recently wrote a fantastic article on this topic. In the article, Haden referenced a group of scientists who theorized that your concept of time is correlated with the amount of new information that comes your way.

When you were younger, you naturally had more first encounters. Do you remember your first kiss, the first day of your first real job or the first time you found out you were pregnant? Of course you do! Not only do you remember the big details, you probably also remember the accompanying sounds, smells, and tastes to boot. Time seemed to halt in those moments. With each "first" your brain makes a new memory template so it can get stored as a robust memory to refer to in case it should happen again.

As you get older, generally there are markedly fewer new experiences and circumstances present in each day. Your brain rapidly processes these familiar daily activities, and therefore, it can feel like time is whizzing by at a faster pace. When things become too familiar, it feels as if time is speeding up.

Could this be a significant ingredient of the average midlife crisis? Generally, there are fewer surprises and new goals to work toward in middle age. We've all heard stories of people in midlife having affairs, leaving great jobs, or buying expensive sports cars. Are they unhappy with their life choices or just really bored with the familiarity of their current circumstances? However, if you find adequate variety in this phase of life, the take home lesson is this: For most women, prioritizing new experiences and adding some novelty into their daily lives is vital for their happiness and fulfillment.

Stay In the Gains

In my late 20s, I fell in love with fiction again after four demanding years of graduate school. I gravitated toward historical fiction books set in faraway lands. One late summer night, I cracked the first page of Arthur Golden's novel *Memoirs of a Geisha*[11] and subsequently lost myself in his mesmerizing story of a young Japanese female entertainer in the first half of the twentieth century.

The full plot evades me today, but I'll never forget his fascinating portrayal of Geisha as a quietly beautiful art form and how its severe precision influenced the culture of Japan during that time. The story beautifully illustrated that when your goal is to get as close to a target as possible, the best way to get there is through small, consistent improvements.

The Japanese call this the philosophy of *kaizen*. *Kaizen* is the idea that little and consistent changes can reap significant improvements. Adopting this mindset, you can feel more motivated to keep growing which, as stated, helps us to stay young at heart and brings more meaning to our days. However, there is one pitfall of *kaizen* to take heed of.

When you devote ample time and energy to self-improvement, it's natural to expect ample results in return. The pitfall is, if you're constantly focused on the distance between you and the finish line, you'll be spending time feeling frustrated in the "I'm not there yet" zone. It's a common trap for women our age. Let me illustrate with a story.

A few years ago, Dr. Brooke and I got the running bug. More accurately, she got the running bug and I came along for the ride. She was training to run a half-marathon with some friends in Raleigh, North Carolina. Not wanting to be left out of a fun girls trip to a cool new city, I nervously registered for the race as well, did a quick Google search and promptly initiated a 12-week running plan. My strategy was to follow this running plan as best as I could and hope for the best.

I started out running one mile and quickly worked up to three miles within a few weeks. I was steadfast but man was it time-consuming! My regular 30-minute weight training sessions were replaced with several hours of running per week. My training peaked at 11 weeks with a nine-mile run. The pride I felt that day is something I'll always cherish.

Race day arrived. We took the obligatory pre-race group photo as our stomachs churned and the nerves set in. None of us had actually run 13.5 miles yet; each of our training guides suggested peaking around nine miles, because running longer can dangerously deplete the body's energy reserves too close to the big day. The shotgun fired and we took our first few steps amid a sea of other runners.

It was slow going at first, but as we worked our way out of the crowd we synced into a pleasant rhythm. Endorphins mixed with the infusion of energy provided by the raucous cheering of the spectators was absolutely intoxicating. I couldn't believe I had made it through the rigors of the last 12 weeks and I felt a sense of pride in my hard work that buoyed me. For quite a few miles, my body felt light as air.

Then around seven miles in, something curious happened. We turned a corner to see two lanes forming ahead of us. We were being corralled—half-marathoners to the left and full marathoners to the right. For the first time since the race began, I focused on the mile marker. It struck me that I was only halfway finished, and it sunk in that those poor souls on the right would have to do my entire run, twice! Here I was feeling pretty good about myself when those guys were about to double me.

Suddenly, my body felt a little heavier. I began to notice the number of inclines far more and the smiling faces on the sidelines far less. The minutes felt like hours. The iTunes playlist I had carefully curated with rhythmic songs designed to match my desired pace seemed to be playing at a breakneck speed. I was so focused on the distance I had yet to run ahead of me that I lost sight of how far I had come. And in those moments, focusing only on what I had yet to achieve, I was miserable.

There is so much beauty in having a compelling vision for your life after kids and also in having some goals in place to help you get there. But it's not achieving the goal alone that will bring you the most happiness. Your vision and goals can be like the horizon—always seeming a little out of reach. When I tell you that you will be happier in life if you take time to look back and measure your success by how far you've come, instead of by how close you are to the finish line, it stems from my own experience.

Dan Sullivan and Benjamin Hardy wrote a book entirely devoted to how to live in the "gains" and stay away from the "gap."[12] It's one of our favorite books we recommend in our community. In addition, a preferred practice of ours to *stay in your gains* is to write down your progress so you can more easily be reminded of how far you've come. I have a unique solution for this.

For more than 10 years (it's never too late or too early to start this practice), I have been jotting down small details on many aspects of my life in a 10-year journal. It consists of one page for each day of the year with each page divided into 10 horizontal sections. Each section is the same day in a different year for 10 years. When I open my 10-year journal and turn to that day's page to make my entry, I'm not only recording my wins and struggles in the last 24 hours but I'm also given a window into the past by reading where I was one year before, all the way back to 10 years ago. It never ceases to amaze me both how much I forget and also *how far I've come.*

It's generally not rereading the big memories that brings me the most satisfaction although that certainly can be fun. For the most part, it's the simple, humdrum details that jump out at me from each page, weaving my life together in front of me like a tapestry. It so clearly shows the full effect and strength of applying daily efforts over time. Have you ever heard the phrase "day by day nothing changes—but in a year everything does." By writing down your daily progress, you'll stay inspired on the days you're feeling defeated about your progress. If you can see your gains more clearly in front of you, you can pat yourself on the back for what you have done and be reminded that continual growth is actually what you're after.

Hobbies Schmobbies

We'd be remiss if we didn't broach the topic of hobbies at some point in this chapter. It's kind of obvious isn't it? Your kids are grown so it's time to get a hobby or a new puppy! If I had a dime every time someone piped up with this advice for struggling empty nester moms on social media, I'd be able to buy a lot of puppies.

So, what's wrong with the advice to get a new hobby? There's nothing wrong per se, but it doesn't account for the inherent differences amid the Four Mom Types. As a Diligent Doer Moms, this advice to "go get a hobby" might actually produce a case of hives because they generally equate hobbies to sitting around breezily painting pottery or whatever else they consider meaningless instead of doing what they really want to do, which is to stay productive.

Let's get on the same page about what defines a hobby. The simple definition of a hobby is an activity that one does for enjoyment, usually without the intent of making a profit. Hobbies differ from passions in that our passions are usually heavily connected to our personal values, whereas hobbies are usually fun, not personal, and not meant to be a stand-in for paid work or for purpose.

Hobbies differ from your purpose in that your purpose is the driving factor that gets you out of bed in the morning, the main vehicle you use to express your passions and your beliefs. Because of the carefree nature by design, hobbies are usually not designed to fill you with a deep sense of accomplishment and mission, but they're a great way to pass a few hours on an otherwise uneventful afternoon. If you are lacking purpose and you're using a hobby to stuff that hole, you might be disappointed. You'd have better luck with that puppy.

Once you've done some work to identify your purpose and your values (refer to Chapter 3 for a refresh) in this phase of life, hobbies can be a great way to round out your lineup. If you're looking for the best ones for you, go back to what you loved as a kid. Hopefully, you have at least one or two activities you did as a child that you looked forward to doing like you looked forward to Christmas. Whatever that thing was, do THAT again. If you enjoyed it as a kid, you might rediscover a love for it again all these years later.

Another way to find your most compatible hobbies is to experiment with as many as you can in a short period of time. If you find an activity that puts you in a flow state, then you've hit the jackpot. A flow state is described as a state of intense concentration. Your focus is so narrow in this state that you shut out all other distractions, and you become completely absorbed by that activity. Because I have ample intrusions in my daily life and information flying at me from all corners, it feels like a breath of fresh air to allow myself to be singularly focused for a few hours of my week.

If you're looking for highly personalized or unique hobby suggestions, we recommend using AI to craft a list of prospective hobbies for you to begin experimenting with. Here's a helpful prompt for you to use in your favorite AI app such as ChatGPT:

> "Please provide a list of hobbies for a woman who has just finished raising her kids. She has ___ hours to spend each week and a budget of _____ dollars to participate each time. Please include both popular and some highly unusual hobbies of women at this age. Consider her fitness level which is beginner/moderate/high/elite."

To take your hobby search up a notch, approach it from the perspective of your Mom type.

- Diligent Doers: Schedule hobby time in your daily schedule or as a to-do to check off. You'll feel better about taking time for a hobby this way.
- Remarkable Relators: Make sure your hobbies include opportunities for connection with others (HINT: Solitary hobbies may not be your thing).

- Awesome Analyzers: Make sure there is plenty of mental stimulation involved. You're more likely to enjoy those hobbies that spark your mental creativity and keep you thinking.
- Magnificent Motivators: You're likely to enjoy competitive pursuits or hobbies that allow you to communicate outwardly (HINT: Silent hobbies may not be your thing).

Remember, your yardstick is growth and learning. Think of those hobbies that allow you to grow and get better physically, emotionally, or cognitively over time. As a reminder, hobbies are designed for fun and generally won't create a new sense of purpose for you. Not all Moms will enjoy or want to take time for hobbies; therefore, hobbies are not obligatory. However, if you do engage, choose hobbies based on how much fun and joy you experience and if you find yourself in a flow state while doing them.

Chapter 12

The Cherry on Top

By Dr. Lynne

There's someone very important in my life who has gone before me to role model what success looks like in this part of life. However, her success may not be obvious at first glance. Before I share more, I'm going to pivot considerably and talk a little smack about Saint Teresa of Calcutta.

Yup, you read that right.

I've always been very intrigued by Mother Teresa. Flashback to Catholic grade school: I sat at my desk in a darkened classroom, watching wide-eyed as a picture of a tiny woman in a blue-bordered sari was projected onto the wall. My 12-year-old brain struggled to match her 76-year-old, frail and crouched exterior with her impressive resume.

At age 69, Mother Theresa won the Nobel Peace Prize. At the time I was studying her, Sister Teresa was still at work, wholly committed to opening new homes for orphans, nursing homes for lepers, and hospices for the terminally ill. She had dedicated her whole life to eradicating the human suffering she found around her.

She was essentially penniless yet she could command millions in just a couple of phone calls. Her influence stretched across the globe. By giving everything she had, she created a legacy that endures today, 28 years after her death, and will likely continue for many years to come.

This was my long-held belief about Mother Teresa. A few years ago, I happened to post a meme on my personal social media page with a beautiful quote from Mother Teresa. Someone I know commented on my post recommending that I Google her. Alluding that there was a dark and controversial side to this devout disciple of Christ, he recommended I research for myself. This was the first time I'd come across anything negative about her. My curiosity was piqued. In the few minutes I spent in the weird and dark section of the Internet that my search took me, I discovered two important things.

The first thing is no matter who you are and how much good you do, you are not immune to criticism and scrutiny. There were a few allegations that Mother Teresa was actually a cruel person and more financially minded than she appeared. I didn't find any credible evidence to support those accusations. This innocent and virtuous woman had been unfairly criticized and targeted by conspiracy theorists in my opinion.

The moral for your life after kids? Be prepared to be criticized or misunderstood by others if you set out to do something bigger, different, or braver than you've ever done. Do it anyway.

Second, there is tremendous, unspoken power in acts of selflessness. It's my personal opinion that Mother Theresa is a righteous example of selflessness: She dedicated her entire being to giving to others and in doing so created a powerful and enduring movement. Putting others' interests ahead of your own doesn't necessarily get rewarded in our culture and it can even be seen as a weakness. I firmly believe that serving others with love and compassion, from a pure desire to be of service to others, foregoing your own gain, takes an incredible amount of self-worth and personal strength.

How exactly does any of this relate to you as a mother in this stage of life? Let me ask you this question: Do you ever feel your kids think the world revolves around them? Your kids have been dependent on you to give them everything they need to survive and grow into healthy and well-adjusted adults. This explains why they are naturally a little selfish. Their brains haven't matured fully yet, and they are busy making sure they get their needs met.

Well, at one time you were their age, too. When you became a parent, in all respects your entire world shifted from being all about you and your needs to caring for the most needy and selfish creature on the planet—the human infant—24 hours a day, seven days a week. Giving to your kids becomes second nature in those early days. It's both a blessing and a curse and following years of giving tirelessly to your kids, naturally many of you feel done with having to give of yourself. At times, you've given more than you had and for some of you there's nothing left to give 18 plus years later.

Despite that fact, finding meaningful ways to give your unique talents to benefit others is a formidable way to find more happiness and fulfillment especially for moms with grown kids.

Betty the Machine

The story I referred to at the start of this chapter is the story of the most selfless and giving Life after Kids mom I know: my own mother, Betty. Our family has affectionately dubbed Betty "the Machine." When I was about 10, I had memories of waking up on a weekend morning, wandering to the bathroom to find my mother on her hands and knees scrubbing every inch of the floor. The floor scrubbing came after she'd set a couple of homemade kneaded loaves of bread in the corner to rise and made a steaming pot of some hearty food—all following her rigorous 40-hour workweek as a cardiovascular nurse.

This was a standard weekend occurrence. Multitasking and working hard to complete tasks are some of her strongest unique abilities. I know, without a doubt, that she never thinks of herself as special. She just does what she does, giving to others first, working hard, and never asking for anything in return, without giving it a thought.

Early in my career, I enlisted my Mom as a guinea pig for more one-on-one coaching experience. She is, as you might have guessed, a Diligent Doer. It wasn't really a surprise to learn that she gets immense satisfaction in being busy and productive. But now I hardly ever question or condemn why she works so hard and won't stop moving.

I've coached other Diligent Doers (including Dr. Brooke) who think there might be something wrong with them at first. They try in vain to relax more and do less, because compared to others they worry they might be too driven. It's usually a relief for them to find out that there's nothing "wrong"—this unique ability to complete tasks is an incredibly powerful and awe-inspiring trait to be embraced and harnessed. In general, the more you know about your strengths the better you can control them, instead of them controlling you.

Betty the Machine is also a Number 2, aka the Helper or the Giver, on the Enneagram. If you recall from Chapter 4, Type 2s are motivated by a strong need to be helpful and giving to others. The strongest wish for Type 2s is to be fully loved and accepted. They often try to get there by being extremely attentive to the needs of those around them and helping other people in any way they can. Knowing what I do about my mom, I think it was especially difficult for her when my sister and I left the house. If you are a Type 2, you may have more difficulty than some other moms and take more time to adapt to your kids leaving.

Quiet Contribution

Our Life after Kids online community is extremely supportive for the most part, but once in a while someone will submit a reply that isn't very kind to a mom who's shared that she's struggling with this transition. The tone of those comments is usually along the lines of "Girl, go get yourself a life."

If you tend to brush off a mom who is having more difficulty than you with the kids growing up, please think about Betty and other Type 2 Moms. They're not only mourning the passing of an era but also the loss of their major reason for being: caring for others. My mom is a stellar example to follow. She thrives by staying busy doing things for us, and she's really in her element when an urgent opportunity to care for someone she loves arises.

When Lila was little, Betty would often visit for a few weeks at a time. She would swoop in, like Mary Poppins, ready to take over and do everything and anything so Mark and I could take a much-needed break. Call me crazy in those days because I would vigorously resist her efforts to help. I was a fledgling mother and homemaker, eager to prove to this woman I admired how capable I was and that I, too, could do it all, without any help. Needless to say, we used to butt heads in those days. Later as I got a little older and frankly more tired, I gave in. When I put my pride aside, I saw how happy it made her to be allowed to step in and help us.

It's obvious to anyone who knows my mom that she doesn't offer to do things for others to gain approval or recognition. She barely expects a thank you. Of course, her efforts do not go unnoticed. Both of my nephews in their 20s are fiercely protective of her and frequently take her to lunch or stop by her house just to see and spend time with her. Her sons-in-law both worship her for lots of reasons but especially because she has always shown her genuine concern for their needs first.

She serves up daily what I've dubbed as *quiet contribution*. She lives alone now that my father has passed, but she still finds purpose in taking care of her younger brother who has health challenges, working part-time as a nurse in a memory care facility, and volunteering at her church and homeless shelter. She loves to dote on her family whenever possible while simultaneously trying not to overstep or overstay her welcome. There are so many women like her out there that are both thoughtful and selfless, but because they contribute so quietly, they will never get the recognition they deserve.

Betty is an outstanding case in point for many of you reading this who simply miss the act of caretaking now that the kids are raised. Each and every one of you should be applauded for your own quiet contribution over the years.

As I've mentioned, my mom doesn't feel she is especially deserving of acknowledgment for doing what comes so easily to her. I feel strongly that people who give of themselves to serve others should never be viewed as doormats or pushovers. Their kindness should never be taken for weakness. On the contrary, in my 50 years of observing my mom, I wholeheartedly see the quiet strength it takes to always put others first time and time again.

As opposed to lacking purpose, which tends to be more about your own self-interests and dreams, lacking ways to give back can also leave us feeling there is something missing. *If you feel some lingering discontent, it's possible it's stemming from having too few opportunities to give of yourself to others in a meaningful way now that you are no longer caring for your family every day.*

I believe in giving attention to both your purpose and the ways you can contribute. Both are healthy and satisfying ways to fill the empty void created by your kids leaving home.

Keep Caretaking, Silly!

I'm terrible at urban slang and Gen Z talk; I sound ridiculous when I say things like "hits different" and "sus," which is short for suspicious in case you're game for learning to talk like a 17-year-old from an old lady. Nevertheless, it's a fun way to embarrass my daughter. She just loves it when I sneak this particular phrase into our conversations: *Players gotta play.*

Players gotta play and moms gotta mom. *If you miss taking care of your kids because they have grown up, moved out, or moved away, find someone else in your life who needs caretaking and give of your time, your heart, and your talents to them.* This is what this next season is all about: Find your strengths and develop ways to give them back to the world. Full stop.

I want to circle back to my earlier point about quiet contributions frequently being mistaken as weakness by others. Some people label those that caretake for others as subservient or submissive. Because of this, you might initially reject the idea of caring for someone other than your children now that they're grown, chalking it up as being beneath you.

I would argue that would be a mistake for many of you. You can get so much meaning, pride, and satisfaction when you do good for others. The more you help others, the more you help yourself in return.

The Brain on Giving Back

If you truly enjoy caring for others, why stop when your kids grow up? However you approach it, finding a way to contribute throughout your life is undoubtedly a method for lifelong happiness and meaning. It's not just beneficial for your emotional health; it's good for your physical health, too.

When we do good for others, our brain responds in a variety of ways. One of the most relevant ways that giving back helps us physically is through the boosting of our brain's production of the neurotransmitters *dopamine* and *serotonin*.

Because these little guys are pretty much running your life, you should probably know a little about them. Much of our behavior in life is determined by the complex reward system that occurs in our brain without us even being aware. We just know if and when we feel good or bad or somewhere in between and often on any given day, all of the above. However, those *feelings* are in large part created by the release of certain brain molecules, in particular dopamine and serotonin, which send signals that directly affect how we feel at any given time.

Serotonin helps to regulate our mood. Large swings in mood are largely attributed to swings in serotonin levels. Sometimes, these swings are medically induced; for instance, a well-known side effect of taking antidepressant medications is a fluctuation of serotonin levels that could result in the very symptoms you are trying to prevent.

Performing good deeds or acts of kindness is scientifically shown to increase serotonin levels in the brain while also reducing cortisol, aka the stress hormone.[9] Similar to a runner's high, there is a phenomenon known as "helper's high" that is basically the result of a rush of serotonin in our brain. Doing good feels good.

As for dopamine, it's most important to know it's the major player when it comes to the reward system in our brain. We become more motivated to repeat certain past behaviors if there is the chance of scoring a dopamine hit even if those behaviors might be potentially harmful to us.

I'm not much of a gambler, but when I visit Las Vegas I make a point to sit down at a slot machine at least once. Ten bets go by and it seems as if all my money is going straight down the drain. But wait . . . on the next spin, as my luck would have it, the fruit and bells align just right and an over-the-top light and sound show starts up, indicating to anyone within 50 feet that I've won. In that moment, my brain receives a nice hit of dopamine. It's widely believed that dopamine plays a significant role in addictions like gambling. Addicts become so intent on chasing the dopamine they get when they win that it's difficult for them to stop even when it's costing them more than they can win back.

Who among us hasn't spent some time mindlessly chasing dopamine even if we didn't know that was the point? For example, endlessly scrolling social media, binge watching TV, overeating junk food, playing addictive video games, or consuming excessive caffeine. All are guaranteed to provide some instant gratification but offer us little to no lasting value. These experiences may feel good for a bit, but they are not good for you to engage in repetitively nor are they good for others.

On the other hand, meaningful activities, such as volunteering, caretaking, or performing random acts of kindness will produce a significant surge of dopamine *and* leave us with lasting satisfaction and feelings of accomplishment afterward. But it's important to acknowledge that these acts may not always feel good in the moment.

If you don't relish the thought of picking up dog poop at your local shelter or entertaining a crabby toddler while her Mom gets a much needed rest, you're not alone. I think it's perfectly okay to admit that. I think this fact is the reason many women are hesitant to seek out these types of experiences at first. But afterward, these types of experiences are not only good for you, they are good for others and they serve the greater good. They give you a boost of dopamine, and they leave you feeling better about yourself and your life than before.

When you start giving back to others, I'm sure that you will immediately notice the difference between "cheap" dopamine thrills and the longer-lasting, more powerful pride in oneself that comes after doing something to make a real difference. My hope is that this conversation will inspire you to try some of these more meaningful activities, elevating your life experience as you contribute your time and talents.

Practical Ways to Contribute

There are a few ways you can determine how to best make your contribution. The first way is to *determine the most urgent and pressing needs in your community and start there.* There are any number of charities and organizations locally and nationally that are desperate for your help. Sometimes, you just need to get started on the wrong thing to eventually lead you to what you are actually meant to do. If you're worried about having enough time or feeling guilted into doing more than you can give right now, remember it's perfectly okay to help out for as little as one hour per week or even just a couple of hours per month. It's also perfectly okay to set a finite time period for your contribution. For example, if you can only volunteer in the spring, let the volunteer coordinator of the charity you select know that you will be only available until the summer starts.

Don't pass up the chance for a life-affirming experience because you've adopted an all or nothing mentality. Some is better than none when it comes to contribution. Even if you wish you could give more, you are more likely to stick with something if you start small and keep your time commitment realistic for you.

The second way is to *find your contribution through your most intense passions*. Our passions are highly personal and emotional for us. They are more likely to spur you to take action because your heart and soul are already so heavily invested. To find your passions, think about what has kept you awake at night in the past. Think about the causes you care about so much that thinking about it causes a visceral response in your body.

For example, whenever I hear about dog or animal mistreatment or abuse, I get an intense physical reaction, which I describe as anger mixed with nausea that sweeps through my entire body. Animal causes are obviously a passion for me. This would be a great place to start in my case.

Another key to your passions can be found in the areas in which we have personally experienced pain or heartache. One of the most powerful and authentic ways to approach your contribution is to get inspired to teach your own personal experience even if it's very painful. I have a friend who endured a rough childhood and who has privately shared that she endured physical and sexual abuse in her household growing up. She has done so much personal work to overcome and transform into the beautiful, loving, and forgiving woman I know her as today. She regularly volunteers at a homeless youth shelter and is often asked to share the things she's done to overcome difficult times for survivor groups. Ironically, because she experienced pain, she can now help free other women from theirs.

Other suggestions to contribute your time and talents to make your contribution are crisis pregnancy centers, domestic abuse shelters, trauma centers, food banks, hospitals, schools, organizations focused on environmental conservation, hospice services, and homeless shelters.

The third method to approach contribution is to *pick ways to contribute by your unique abilities.* Let me give a few examples so you can understand what I mean by this. I have a friend, Heather, who is a Type 1 on the Enneagram, which if you recall is also known as the Perfectionist. She has a knack for organizing, beautifying, and simplifying spaces because she naturally spots the imperfections in her environment and like a heat-seeking missile she can't rest until she can fix it by making it "perfect" again. As you can imagine, Heather's home is aesthetically beautiful and well organized. But she also chooses to apply these talents through contribution. Each year at Thanksgiving she visits a shelter for women and children seeking safety from domestic abuse, along with her kids, to volunteer for the holiday. While the rest of her family serves a meal, she sets her sights on the shelter's pantry, which at Thanksgiving time is usually overflowing with new donations. It's a good problem for the pantry that people are dropping off donations faster than they can be sorted and shelved; nevertheless, that disorganization makes it hard for the staff to find what they need.

This is where Heather shines. She goes to work, and when she's finished unboxing, sorting, and organizing, everything is in its rightful place and order is restored to the pantry again. My ear is always listening for stories like this. When Heather first told me about her shelter work, we were having coffee. I asked her some questions, excited that she had found something so perfectly suited for her that was helping others. I praised her for her efforts, but she leaned in and with a sheepish look she said, "Actually Lynne, I feel guilty that it's pretty enjoyable for me. Cleaning and organizing is my favorite thing in the whole world; you know that." She played it off like it was no big deal, but all I could think was how cool it is that she's found a way to give back that's also so fun and joyful for her.

I have another bestie who is a Type 5 on the Enneagram. Fives are typically known as the Investigators, they have a knack for academic pursuits, are often subject matter experts, and are usually curious people but sometimes have difficulty showing emotion. My friend is super smart and mega-insightful. She has started volunteering for a local artistic collective helping to balance their accounts and advise on expenditures. She, too, loves her volunteer work and now that her kids are older, she's found it gives her something to look forward to each week. Giving back can be surprisingly fun and thoroughly enjoyable if it also falls within your personal zone of genius. In both of these examples, these ladies would probably tell you that they are getting far more from giving back than they would have thought possible.

Dr. Brooke and I discuss this topic on the podcast frequently. You can listen to the full episodes wherever you listen to podcasts, but here's a summary list to get you started.

- Type 1, *The Perfectionist*: Efficiency is what you do well. Let the charities you volunteer for know that you like organizing, decorating, and creating systems for bringing more ease to their patrons and staff. Or find a busy Mom friend or neighbor who could use your talents to make her life more organized and offer to help in her home.

- Type 2, *The Helper*: Giving back to others comes so easily to you. Think of families in your circle who could benefit from your natural caretaking abilities and offer to help them. Wherever possible, apply your time where caring for people or animals is the goal. Strategic behind-the-scenes work likely won't carry the same appeal for you as would spending time on the frontlines with the very people you wish to help.

- Type 3, *The Performer*: Results are your jam so stick to activities that will produce a tangible outcome. Building a house for a deserving family from start to finish is one example. You may be attracted to public relations work or speaking on behalf of a charity as well.

- Type 4, *The Individualist*: You are generally sensitive to emotions so performing big and small acts of meaningful work for marginalized populations is particularly attractive for Type 4s. Knowing your work carries meaning is the key. Bonus points if it's unusual or uncommon work—you prefer to be different.

- Type 5, *The Investigator*: Your thoughtful and well-researched approach is your superpower. Serving as an advisor on a charity board can be a good alignment for Type 5s. Behind the scenes bookwork or auditing is also generally in your lane. Something related to working with numbers or behind the scenes developing strategies are two examples of probable agreeable alignment for 5s.

- Type 6, *The Loyalist*: Engage with charities that align with your passions at heart. You may find yourself preferring to restrict your efforts to one or two charities that you return to for predictable work you can perform regularly. In general, you're a model contributor for any charity because you are so dependable and loyal.

- Type 7, *The Enthusiast*: Variety and adventure is a perfect combination for giving back for Type 7s. Don't restrict yourself to just one charity; feel free to explore and give in many places. Short-term stints are great for you—volunteering at charity concerts or races are an example. You can be especially useful when it comes to planning "the fun" in a fundraising effort.

- Type 8, *The Challenger*: You are well-suited for high-intensity situations, so you may find yourself attracted to difficult tasks that others may not be cut out for. You have the required tough exterior to handle grueling jobs, like on the ground rescue attempts or mitigating inhumane environments. Acting as a lead advocate, whether it's asking for funds or leading a fund-raising committee, is also in your wheelhouse.

- Type 9, *The Peacemaker*: Working within a team of committed individuals to bring about change is a great contribution scenario for Type 9s. You generally fit in well and provide the glue that keeps the group together, which helps to maximize synergy in group efforts.

Pay attention when a cause or problem in the world speaks to your sensibilities—that's your nudge to get involved in some way. Remember that making a real difference in the areas that you care most about, however small or big, is about as satisfying and fulfilling as it gets.

Conclusion

By Dr. Brooke

As Lynne mentioned, I am indeed an Enneagram Type 6, and she's right when she says that as a 6, my favorite ways to contribute are supporting charities that I feel passionately about.

For me, everything I know about donating money, my time, or my talents came from my parents, not because they told me what to do, but because they showed me by the way they lived. For instance, during the holidays, our home was always open to people that had no place to go or not enough money to celebrate.

One year, my dad took me with him to a patient's home for a very special Christmas Eve surprise that I will never forget. We went to the home of a single mom who was barely getting by and unable to give her young son a proper Christmas. She had no idea we were coming, so imagine her surprise when we showed up at her house with a sack full of treasures that included the most sought after gift of the year, a Nintendo game console, explaining to her bright-eyed little boy that Santa had stopped by our house earlier that day asking if we would do him a favor and drop off the presents because he was just so busy that year. As long as I live, I'll never forget the look of pure joy on that little boy's face and the tears of happiness streaming from his mother's eyes.

Take it from me and my dad, contributing to the world and helping people and organizations in your community is one of the best gifts you can give to yourself in this phase of life especially if you're seeking more meaning and fulfillment. But let's not miss the other important lesson from my parents because, if you notice, I said earlier that everything I know about contribution I learned from them. This confirms what I mentioned in a previous chapter about our kids learning more from what we do than what we say. And yes, regardless of their age or ours, they are still learning from us today. We never stop mothering.

Until now, this book has focused on you, not your kids, because your purpose and happiness in this phase of life should not come solely from them. For true and lasting happiness, you have to find purpose and fulfillment apart from your kids after they are grown. And yet, in a surprising turn of events, your kids are actually a very important part to rediscovering yourself and thriving beyond motherhood. Here's why.

We know that you, like us, love your kids more than you love yourself. And we know that sometimes you need a bigger "why" beyond yourself to create change and improve your life. So, if you've come this far and you're struggling to get motivated to take action or you're feeling overwhelmed at the thought of implementation, think about your kids.

If you aren't yet prepared to live a more meaningful life now that they're grown for yourself, do it for them because your kids are still watching everything you do. And every time you take steps to find more purpose, get to know yourself better, manage stress and your emotions more appropriately, improve your physical fitness, or cultivate beauty in your life and get comfortable in your own skin, they see you. When you make connections, forge a stronger community, build deeper friendships, push yourself out of your comfort zone, or learn something new, they watch and learn.

Of course, every time you give back they believe that they, too, can make a difference in the world. Our kids are still learning how to do life and how to believe in themselves and they're taught, at least in part, by watching how we do our lives and believe in ourselves. So, let today be the first day of the rest of your very meaningful and fulfilling life after kids, and give your children the gift of knowing that anything is possible, goals are attainable, and dreams do come true.

References

1. Vaillant, G. E., McArthur, C. C., and Bock, A. "Grant Study of Adult Development, 1938–2000" (2022). https://doi.org/10.7910/DVN/48WRX9, Harvard Dataverse, V4, UNF:6:FfCNPD1m9jk950Aomsriyg== [fileUNF].
2. Mayo Clinic Staff, "Friendships: Enrich your Life and Improve your Health," 15 October 2024. https://www.mayoclinic.org/healthy-lifestyle/adult-health/in-depth/friendships/art-20044860.
3. Clifton, D. *Now, Discover Your Strengths*. Free Press, 2001.
4. Gallup. "Clifton StrengthsFinder Assessment." https://store.gallup.com/h/en-us.
5. Rath, T. *StrengthsFinder 2.0*. Gallup Press, 2007.
6. Cron, I.M. and Stabile, S. *The Road Back to You*. InterVarsity Press, 2016.
7. Holt-Lunstad, J., Smith, T. B., and Layton, J. B. "Social Relationships and Mortality Risk: A Meta-Analytic Review." *PLOS Medicine* 7, no. 7(2010): e1000316. https://doi.org/10.1371/journal.pmed.1000316.

8. Smith, C. "How Social Connection Supports Longevity." Stanford Center on Longevity, 18 December 2023. https://longevity.stanford.edu/lifestyle/2023/12/18/how-social-connection-supports-longevity/.

9. Cain, S. *Quiet: The Power of Introverts in a World That Can't Stop Talking.* Random House, 2012.

10. Manly, J. J., Jones, R. N., Langa, K. M., et al. "Estimating the Prevalence of Dementia and Mild Cognitive Impairment in the US: The 2016 Health and Retirement Study Harmonized Cognitive Assessment Protocol Project." *JAMA Neurology* 79, no. 12 (2022): 1242–1249. https://doi.org/10.1001/jamaneurol.2022.3543.

11. Haden, J. "Want to Feel You're Living a Longer and Fuller Life? Neuroscience Says Making Denser Memories Is the Best Way to Slow the Passage of Time." *Inc. Magazine*, 15 August 2024.

12. Golden, A. *Memoirs of a Geisha.* Alfred A. Knopf, 1997.

13. Hardy, B., and Sullivan, D. *The Gap and the Gain.* Hay House, 2021.

14. Lynn University. "Why Doing Good Feels So Good," 13 February 2017. https://www.lynn.edu/news/2017/why-doing-good-feels-so-good.